Volunteering in Global Mental Health

Volunteering in Global Mental Health

A Practical Guide for Clinicians

Edited by

Sophie Thomson
World Psychiatric Association

Peter Hughes
Springfield University Hospital, London

Sam Gnanapragasam
South London and Maudsley NHS Foundation Trust

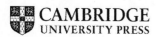

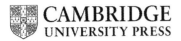

Shaftesbury Road, Cambridge CB2 8EA, United Kingdom

One Liberty Plaza, 20th Floor, New York, NY 10006, USA

477 Williamstown Road, Port Melbourne, VIC 3207, Australia

314–321, 3rd Floor, Plot 3, Splendor Forum, Jasola District Centre, New Delhi – 110025, India

103 Penang Road, #05–06/07, Visioncrest Commercial, Singapore 238467

Cambridge University Press is part of Cambridge University Press & Assessment, a department of the University of Cambridge.

We share the University's mission to contribute to society through the pursuit of education, learning and research at the highest international levels of excellence.

www.cambridge.org
Information on this title: www.cambridge.org/9781108827003

DOI: 10.1017/9781108920728

First published 2023

A catalogue record for this publication is available from the British Library.

A Cataloging-in-Publication data record for this book is available from the Library of Congress

ISBN 978-1-108-82700-3 Paperback

Cambridge University Press & Assessment has no responsibility for the persistence or accuracy of URLs for external or third-party internet websites referred to in this publication and does not guarantee that any content on such websites is, or will remain, accurate or appropriate.

....

Every effort has been made in preparing this book to provide accurate and up-to-date information that is in accord with accepted standards and practice at the time of publication. Although case histories are drawn from actual cases, every effort has been made to disguise the identities of the individuals involved. Nevertheless, the authors, editors, and publishers can make no warranties that the information contained herein is totally free from error, not least because clinical standards are constantly changing through research and regulation. The authors, editors, and publishers therefore disclaim all liability for direct or consequential damages resulting from the use of material contained in this book. Readers are strongly advised to pay careful attention to information provided by the manufacturer of any drugs or equipment that they plan to use.

Contents

Section 4 Future of Global Volunteering

Foreword

The editors have brought together their own and others' experiences of volunteering over the past 15 years in a practical manual designed to support people who want to join the ranks of volunteers in the future. They hope that the historical brain drain of professionals from low- and middle-income countries to the UK could be reversed with more UK-trained mental health professionals supporting the development of services through training projects internationally, both with remote and face-to-face partnerships. Stories from volunteers in this book consistently report learning a great deal themselves as well as often having profound personal experiences.

The word 'transformative' repeats in the accounts of the lived experiences of volunteers. Most of the volunteers' stories have the following in common:

- taking a leap into a new world armed with goodwill, good preparation and some courage
- adapting to new cultures demanding flexibility and an open mind
- being grateful for all that is offered with humility and honesty
- living away from familiar supports allowing for reflection on what is really important
- finding as a welcome surprise personal resources and skills previously unexplored

My own experience of international volunteering started by working with Voluntary Service Overseas (VSO) in Nigeria as a young woman. I experienced first-hand the value of volunteering and this helped me to persist with developing international work throughout my career.

As a member of the Board of International Affairs at the Royal College of Psychiatrists, I explored the different options open to the College, including trialling a VSO-led programme for trainee psychiatrists. There were quite a few hurdles to overcome for the College to establish and run its own volunteer programme, including resistance from some in the College but particularly the need for a start-up fund. I arranged a fundraising trek in India for a week, which ended with a visit to mental health services in Kerala.

As president of the Royal College of Psychiatrists, some of my proudest moments were visiting all of our six international divisions, testament to the College's large international membership of psychiatrists who had trained in the UK. Some of course had stayed and made invaluable contributions to mental health services in the United Kingdom. On a visit to Northern Pakistan in 2007 to attend a World Psychiatric Association (WPA) regional meeting, I was surprised to learn that there were around 350 psychiatrists in the whole of Pakistan but, at the same time, a similar number of Pakistani psychiatrists were working in the UK. Many of the latter returned to their home country regularly to visit family and friends and often to share their skills and resources too. One such person was Dr Afzal Javed, now president of the WPA. In 2007, Dr Javed arranged a tour for myself and colleagues to visit earthquake-stricken parts of Northern Pakistan, including meetings with senior government ministers, the National Mental Health Taskforce, international development agencies as well as academic and other leading psychiatrists to think about their mental health response. When the earthquake happened in 2005, very large numbers of children had been bereaved and traumatised, but there were no mental health services available to them or to those supporting them. A child psychiatrist from North London volunteered to spend a year in Rawalpindi training and mentoring local psychiatrists and health workers to reach out to these children. I remember conversations with this volunteer's medical director in North London to support her requested period of unpaid leave, and on her return to enable her to continue her mentoring role remotely. There were three or four other year-long placements around this time to other countries too. Another success was signing a MOU (memorandum of understanding) with the Iraqi regional government in Kurdistan to deliver some training in Iraq.

In 2009, in a memo to my successor as president, who was considering outsourcing the programme, I advised that:

> 'the unique aspect of the College programme is its ability to respond to requests from members for a particular technical support or training, and /or to support diaspora members to make a sustainable and targeted contribution in their home country. I see it primarily as being a service to our overseas members. This is what distinguishes it from any other agencies' volunteer programmes.'

Projects have been undertaken in highly challenging contexts such as Iraq and Myanmar as well as in Malawi, Ghana and elsewhere, supported as needed by the Volunteering and International Psychiatry Special Interest Group (VIPSIG). At the time of writing, a growing number of College members and other mental health professionals are donating their time to mental health and intellectual disability services in low- and middle-income countries, with VIPSIG hoping that the programme will grow to support 100 volunteers annually. Of course, the pandemic may have changed some of our ideas about how training and volunteering can best be offered. For example, does volunteering still necessarily involve travelling? By empowering people from afar and helping people to adapt ideas for their own culture, their own organisational reality may prove as or more effective. And the wider availability of mobile technology to provide virtual supervision/consultation and our growing familiarity with webinars and hybrid conferences changes a lot.

Having been part of getting the volunteer programme at The Royal College of Psychiatrists off the ground, I am thrilled to read that volunteering is now an integral part of the College's international strategy. This is entirely due to the energy and commitment of so many people, either as volunteers themselves or as leaders who have been determined to develop a sustainable College led volunteer scheme.

In this book you will read about how to prepare and carry out volunteering and training internationally as well as how best to support service development. This is brought to life by hearing inspirational stories from several volunteers about their own unique experiences of volunteering. A common theme is the realisation of how much a volunteer brings back to their everyday work. As one volunteer said: 'I certainly learnt as much, if not more, than I taught' – a sentiment that many volunteers share. I hope you will be inspired to join the global community of volunteers and to encourage others to volunteer too.

Professor Sheila the Baroness Hollins

Contributors

Name	Title	Given Affiliation	Degrees
Sophie Thomson	Dr	World Psychiatric Association Co-Chair Volunteering Working Group Retired NHS Consultant Psychiatrist	MRCP, MRCPsych
Peter Hughes	Dr	Retired NHS Consultant Psychiatrist Southwest London and St George's Mental Health NHS Trust Independent MHPSS Consultant	MB BAO Bch, MSc, FRCPsyc
Sam Gnanapragasam	Dr	Wellcome CREATE PhD Fellow Institute of Psychiatry, Psychology & Neuroscience, King's College London and Specialty Registrar in Psychiatry South London and Maudsley NHS Foundation Trust	BSc, MBBS, MRCPsych
Ayesha Ahmad	Dr	Reader in Global Health Humanities St George's University of London	PhD
Bradley Hillier	Dr	Consultant Forensic Psychiatrist, West London NHS Trust	BMBCh, MA(Oxon), MFFLM, FRCPsych

(cont.)

Name	Title	Given Affiliation	Degrees
Dinesh Bhugra	Professor	Professor Emeritus, Centre for Affective Disorders, Institute of Psychiatry, Psychology & Neuroscience, King's College London	MA, MSc, FRCP, FRCPE, FRCPsych, PhD
Sai Kham Thaw	Dr	Medical Support Worker London Northwest University Healthcare NHS Trust and Mind to Mind Myanmar	MBBS, MS
Djibril Ibrahim Moussa Handuleh	Dr	Psychiatrist, Amoud University, Borama, Somaliland	
Mandip Jheeta	Dr	Consultant Forensic Psychiatrist Barnet, Enfield and Haringey Mental Health NHS Trust	MRCPsych
Dorcas Gwata	Ms	Mental Health Nurse and Independent Global Health Consultant	MSc
Anna Walder	Dr	Psychiatrist, previously South London and Maudsley NHS Foundation Trust	MRCPsych
Jane Mounty	Dr	Retired Consultant Psychiatrist	MRCPsych
Sally Browning	Dr	Retired Consultant in Adult General Psychiatry Oxleas NHS Foundation Trust, 1988–2009	MRCPsych

(cont.)

Name	Title	Given Affiliation	Degrees
Ruairi Page	Dr	Consultant Forensic Psychiatrist HMP Dovegate, HMP Hewell, HMP Featherstone Midlands Partnership NHS Foundation Trust St George's Hospital	MRCPsych
Dawn Harris	Dr	Psychiatrist, Devon Partnership NHS Trust	MBBCh, MRCPsych

Introduction

Sophie Thomson, Peter Hughes and Sam Gnanapragasam

For most, if not all, volunteers, the experience of volunteering globally is a professional and personal highlight. It changes volunteers as mental health professionals and as people. Many of the experiences outlined in this book have been transformative. For those fortunate enough to join professional colleagues in other countries, there are opportunities to learn to see beyond a narrow medical perspective into a broader socio-cultural canvas, especially when working with the limited resources available in many countries. Multiple skills may be needed, and volunteers can expand their repertoire of skills in service development, supervision, teaching and cultural awareness. Encounters with new challenges, resource difficulties and obstacles can help with working practices upon return to the NHS. Volunteering can be unsuccessful as well as successful and this book is about maximising success. The book attempts to demonstrate ways to become a more culturally competent and skilled mental health professional through global volunteer work.

People volunteer at different stages of their careers, from student days to post retirement. The reasons are varied, but common motivations include altruism and the desire to 'give something back'. Many readers may wish to contribute to the welfare of people overseas with mental illness, alongside some who feel a deep desire to do what they can for those who have little access to mental health care. For people from a diaspora background, there may be a desire to help 'back home'. For others, it is motivated by a need for refreshment and to gain new perspectives away from the usual daily professional ways of working. Some may feel the desire to contribute to colleagues' development or make an impact on trainees and the next generation. Other volunteers may crave ethical travel, and some mention the increasing appeal of learning from colleagues in varied and low resource settings. Whatever the reason(s), careful ethical reflection is indeed needed as outlined in Chapters 3 and 4 on ethical consideration.

This book seeks to help prospective volunteers feel more informed, better prepared and inspired to be effective and ethical volunteers. It outlines key principles and practicalities to consider. This book is not intended to be viewed or read from cover to cover as an academic text. Instead, it seeks to be an evidence-based practical guide that readers can interact with depending on their specific interests and needs. It is based on up-to-date evidence in global mental health and the experiences of the authors (which includes both volunteers and those in host countries who are the recipients of voluntary projects). Emphasis is placed on global volunteering undertaken through partnership models of cooperative working with international colleagues.

The book is written with mental health professionals in mind: doctors, nurses, psychologists and other therapists, but we also hope it will be useful for other professionals including those working in social care, students and health-allied volunteers. It is written to be accessible to all career stages. Although the book is primarily structured for UK-based clinicians (with use of related nomenclature), it is hoped that it will have a resonance for an international audience outside of the UK and be of help to those involved in other global volunteering partnerships, including South-South projects. To aid this, definitions of UK-specific nomenclature are contextualised and defined in the appendix.

Key Considerations

Global volunteering can initially be seen as a very simple transaction, but it is actually quite complex and requires purposeful consideration. This section outlines key considerations that the reader should take into account when navigating global mental health volunteering.

Global Mental Health Context

There are huge inequalities around the world in the provision of care for people with mental health difficulties. The gap between need and the provision of services for people with mental health illness is very large indeed, especially in low- and middle-income countries (LMICs)[1]. People with mental illness face stigma, violation of human rights and poverty in many parts of the world. To ensure that those suffering from mental illnesses are neither ignored nor forgotten, there is a need to foster a public mental health approach and help build health system capacity.

The effects of social determinants such as absolute poverty can be particularly prominent in LMICs. Also, volunteers need to be alert to considerations such as gender-based violence, child protection and vulnerable groups. The issues raised can be as varied as social inclusion, confidentiality and different forms of abuse. Prospective volunteers need to be well-informed on matters of human rights, which are a fundamental pillar on which modern global volunteering is now built. Mentally ill and intellectually disabled people are at particular risk of violations of their human rights. This can be a complex area where the volunteer may well need advice, support and supervision. The Royal College of Psychiatrists has a Committee on Human Rights and this group, in addition to the host country's ethics institutions and colleagues, can be a source of informed advice.

Mutual Learning and Partnership Working

Volunteering to work overseas, particularly in LMICs, has a great deal to teach us. Professionals in high-income countries, including the UK, must guard against promoting 'medical imperialism', by which is meant that only we have the 'right approach' and that we know best. Attitudes of this kind get in the way of progress and are harmful to making a mutually beneficial relationship where everyone both learns and teaches.

Volunteering is about co-production and partnership. Any volunteering should come after a request from a host country and not something clinicians in the United Kingdom 'do' to other countries. As volunteers are guests, there is a need to demonstrate appropriate humility. Volunteering should be in the context of sustainable programmes and skills transfer.

Although many countries have historically adopted Western models of assessment and treatment of mental disorders, there have also been creative and innovative solutions to serve the needs of people in LMICs. We have much to learn from our colleagues overseas; for example, the use of *The Friendship Bench* in rural Zimbabwe communities[2]. In this project, brief training in basic counselling is given to appropriate community members who can then offer psychological support in problem-solving at the community level. It has been shown to be successful in managing common mental health difficulties and has now been adopted in other countries. Mindfulness too has global roots. Partnership is key – it is a two-way learning and participatory approach.

Flexibility and Attention to Assessed Needs

The mainstay of partnership working is currently the development of mutually agreed training programmes. However, other needs may be identified, and volunteers may be asked to carry out different tasks, from organising written protocols and academic curricula, to helping with team development, supervising clinical work, public health messaging, the promotion of mental health awareness and so many other opportunities. It is important that a volunteer is flexible and responsive to the needs and requests of the local partners. There may be times when you may feel out of your depth, or that you do not yet have the skills necessary for the required tasks. In those circumstances, it is necessary to be transparent with your local partners and problem-solve together.

Knowledge and Skills Required

Psychiatrists and other mental health volunteers will probably need to go beyond their habitual professional comfort zones. Before working with international colleagues, volunteers usually need to refresh their own knowledge and skills across a wide range of mental health topics, including basic principles of care and mental health assessment and management. Thankfully there are some really helpful resources becoming available about working internationally, some of which are listed at the end of the book (see Appendix 1). International volunteers may find themselves covering mental health care for persons of all ages from child to old age and competence may be required in areas such as drug and alcohol misuse and developmental and organic disorders.

Organic disorders presenting as mental illnesses are more common in LMICs as the burden of TB, HIV, other infectious disorders, head injury and epilepsy is much higher. In fact, epilepsy is now included in many WHO mental health-related training materials, including the WHO mhGAP (Mental Health Gap Action Programme)[3]. This includes mhGAP Intervention Guide – Version 2 which a training manual of integrating mental health into primary care that is discussed throughout this book[4]. Primary care volunteers and psychiatrists offering training for colleagues wanting to enhance local primary care skills may find this particularly beneficial.

Working with all people involved in the provision of health and mental health services helps spread awareness, improves skills for everyone and can challenge stigmatisation. One of the many skills that volunteers can learn from working internationally is the value of public mental health messaging and advocacy. Engaging managers, local officials and academics, local non-government organisations (NGOs) and other stakeholders substantially supports the sustainability of projects. It can feel overwhelming even to think about how to develop services, but as mental health professional trainers, it is important to include clinicians in service development projects. In the chapters on the lived experiences of recent volunteers, there are examples of creative and practical ways to enhance training with attention to opportunities to advocate for changes that make a lasting impact.

Experience suggests that people who enjoy successful volunteering experiences with international colleagues usually:

- Know enough up-to-date evidence-based basic psychiatry (or their speciality) and are able to adapt their knowledge to new settings in a way that respects culture
- Enjoy teaching and learning
- Communicate well with colleagues from other cultures and enjoy working creatively and flexibly with new acquaintances
- Behave professionally, with respect, courtesy, honesty and humility
- Are ready to face challenges, be solution-focused and are prepared to manage outside their comfort zone
- Are emotionally mature and tolerate uncertainty and the '"grey areas'

Professionalism

Unpaid work in another country requires the same level of professional behaviour, preparation, ongoing training and supervision as paid work. For volunteering to be impactful and professional, it needs to be carefully planned and based on available evidence, mutual respect between colleagues and appropriate support and self-care.

Awareness of Settings, Environment and Safety

Personal safety is an important and common concern for volunteers visiting other countries. It is important to get advice from host countries, and the UK Foreign, Commonwealth & Development Office (FCDO) travel advice should always be adhered to[5]. The FCDO has regularly updated, helpful and reliable information on safety and possible dangers. However, even if the FCDO says that most visits are trouble-free, all travellers, but especially inexperienced travellers, would be wise to keep alert and follow a risk assessment process, and to avoid travelling alone if at all possible. The personal health and safety of oneself as well as colleagues based in other countries can sometimes be an important factor in successfully settling into the practicalities of working in a new environment, and support and supervision may be needed.

Difficult Political Environments

One of the challenges of working in countries with known governmental violations of human rights is finding a way to separate the volunteering work from the government or organisations who are abusing their power. Many charities and international organisations manage to make it clear that providing assistance neither condones nor supports the actions of the government in the country where they are working.

Careers in Global Mental Health

A career path for global mental health is beginning to take shape. There are opportunities in the United Nations (UN), UN-related organisations such as the World Health Organization (WHO) and NGOs based in different countries. For some of these roles, it is necessary to have a postgraduate master's or PhD degree in public or global health. A diploma in tropical medicine is also welcomed. People in this career need to be prepared to change jobs relatively frequently and move between different countries. At the same time, being grounded and having a home base is also important.

Experience as a volunteer can sometimes assist in accessing courses and jobs internationally. Volunteering may also help people find out whether living and working internationally will really work out as a suitable career choice. Experience in volunteering adds to one's CV and volunteers often comment that it is frequently the liveliest part of their job interviews.

Finance and Money

Generally, volunteer work is not well-funded, but those people generous enough to volunteer their time and skills should not need to be paying for their own transportation and accommodation. Ideally good projects involve the host organisations paying for and arranging accommodation, transfers and a training venue in the country.

For short projects, volunteers working in the NHS have, historically, taken study leave or unpaid leave. This could change, but the current economic climate suggests that volunteers should anticipate paying for some expenses. Some volunteers think of this as a contribution to charity and to their own development.

Personal Benefit and Gain

Volunteering can undoubtedly help open one's mind to other ways of working with the clinical and educational challenges which we all face today. It can also be worth recognising that placements can add colour to your CV, in addition to helping develop new skills and enhance existing knowledge.

Limitations Related to Staffing Numbers and Global Recruitment Practices

It is important to be mindful that there are limitations on the impact that volunteers can make in some contexts, particularly given inequalities in health and wealth globally. This is clear when we consider the number of health staff available and working in different parts of the world:

- An estimated shortage of 43 million health workers in 2019 globally (6.4 million doctors, 30.6 million nurses/midwives, 3.3 million dentistry personnel and 2.9 million pharmaceutical personnel) relative to the workforce needed to provide universal health coverage[6].
- A workforce unevenly spread, with high-income countries having 115 per 10,000 population of nurses/midwives whereas low-income countries have an average of 9 nurses/midwives per 10,000[7].

This phenomenon is further exacerbated by the process of high-income countries, including the United Kingdom, recruiting health personnel (including in mental health) to fill domestic gaps. An estimated 15% of health workers globally are from countries outside of their birth or from where they achieved their professional qualification[8].

Global volunteering, in the current model, does not address this directly. Whilst focus on training can help build capacity, there is a need for 'beyond volunteering' approaches focused on advocacy domestically to ensure policy and practice is ethical. Indeed, the system of recruitment needs justice not charity to ensure that there is not a greater brain drain and that we are able to build better health systems globally in a sustainable manner.

Part of understanding limitations and tackling such practice is recognising the different power relationships between high-income and other countries, and their organisations and projects. It is worth a prospective volunteer being versed in the increasing literature related to education, training, health and international affairs around decolonisation and ensuring parity of power, decision-making and relationship building.

Volunteering Locally in the United Kingdom

It is important to recognise the considerable value to the development of skills that can be gained through volunteering in the United Kingdom.

Indeed, documenting the details of all the volunteering work undertaken within the UK would produce a very full book indeed. However, as this is beyond the scope of this book, there is limited discussion related to these opportunities. The Volunteering and International Psychiatry Special Interest Group of the Royal College of Psychiatrists (VIPSIG) knows from its annual essay prize that students are promoting mental health awareness as well as volunteering their time in all sorts of creative ways. Volunteers are teaching in religious institutions including churches and mosques, whilst many psychiatrists, senior and junior, give their time to societies and charities ranging from sporting clubs to groups such as Medical Justice.

As an example, Medical Justice welcomes health professional volunteers to visit detainees in detention and write reports and provide opinions. 'By joining Medical Justice, health professionals can have a positive impact on the lives and health of this most vulnerable group of people in the UK'[9]. Mental health professionals have also volunteered to work with the UK Refugee Council in a variety of ways, especially over the past few years when so many asylum seekers and refugees have been moving across Europe and seeking refuge in the United Kingdom.

There have been so many more acts of kindness and sharing of expertise, especially during the Covid pandemic. Perhaps many of these volunteers have experienced the satisfaction of voluntary work and want to do more. National and international volunteering has become more straightforward now that electronic resources are being developed and we can work in new ways with colleagues anywhere in the world from our own homes.

Conclusion

In reading this book, including the first-hand narrative experiences of a number of volunteers and host recipients, it is hoped that you will feel more prepared, confident and inspired to take your next step in global volunteering. The voluntary placement can take many shapes and sizes. Your placement may be a short- or longer-term one, be based in places where the spoken language is shared or varied, and your day-to-day role may be primary training, teaching, supervising, researching, project managing, capacity building and/or more. The rewards of these placements can be outstanding and transformative for many, both personally and professionally. As a prospective volunteer, we hope that the information contained within this book will give you some additional confidence to jump in and begin to be part of developing a more equitable, ethical and sustainable global mental health voluntary community.

What Is in the Book

The book makes suggestions on negotiating the practicalities of getting from an initial interest in volunteering to the completion of a successful project and safe return home. It is not an exhaustive summary of all possible opportunities and experiences but rather hopes to give a range of representative experiences and advice that inspire, stimulate and enable reflection for the reader.

The book is organised in **four sections** – the theoretical and practical considerations outlined in Sections 1 and 2 are complemented by the rich narrative accounts and experiences of volunteers in Section 3. Section 4 looks to the future with an exploration of electronic learning and reflections on what might happen next as global mental health voluntary work gathers pace.

The book begins with a **review of principles and theory** in global volunteering. Herein, Chapter 1 introduces the field of global mental health and the notable theoretical principles to be considered. This includes a review of documents such as the Lancet series on Global Mental Health, the WHO World Mental Health Action Plan and mental health law as well as training delivery tools such as the WHO Mental Health Gap Action Programme (mhGAP)[3]. There is then a focused chapter on **humanitarian settings** with both theoretical as well as practical considerations (Chapter 2). Principles in humanitarian emergency response include preparedness, the need for multi-sectoral response, 'building back better', the role of co-ordination, the prioritisation of safety and the necessity for situational and needs analysis. Key humanitarian tools are introduced including the Inter-Agency Standing Committee (IASC)[10] and SPHERE[11] guidelines. The chapter emphasises that no one should volunteer in isolation, and it is important to be part of a responsible and sustainable programme.

Chapters 3 and 4 then consider **key ethical and cultural principles** about global volunteering, including discussions of case studies involving challenging ethical scenarios. Finally, this section concludes with a discussion around the **benefits of volunteering for the trainee and the UK health system** (Chapter 5). This discussion demonstrates that global volunteering can be a win-win opportunity that enhances not only the skills and knowledge of the international community but also brings considerable benefits after return to the UK, including enhanced teaching and clinical skills, leadership capability and cultural awareness.

The second section is a **practical guide and toolkit** to support global volunteering. The chapters in this section are focused on practical considerations related to preparation, on-site working and project delivery, training, monitoring and evaluation, and post-trip sustainability. Chapter 6 on **preparation** considers careful planning with host partners, and tips to enable living and working safely in another country. The **'on the ground' considerations,** particularly cultural understanding and respect upon arrival, are considered in Chapter 7.

Chapter 8 on **implementing and delivering training** describes how a passion for teaching and learning, especially with confidence in the creative use of interactive teaching techniques, brings the training experience to life and can make it enjoyable for all. The following Chapter 9 introduces a **new psychological toolkit** with simple psychological interventions suitable for all professionals. There is then an exploration of what happens after a global volunteering trip, with an examination of the process of **coming home, supervision, sustainable practice and self-care** (Chapter 10). This reiterates the importance of careful preparation throughout an entire project. Finally, this section concludes by considering the necessary steps in **monitoring and evaluation** and emphasises the need to ensure that metrics are developed with and owned by local partners (Chapter 11).

In the third section, narrative accounts provide rich **reflective perspectives on global volunteering.** There are narratives from the recipients of volunteer workers as well as global health volunteers giving varied accounts of their lived experiences. Some of these experiences relate to capacity building, humanitarian work, delivering training, receiving training and providing supervision. Some are about short trips and others extend over years. Most involve training and raising awareness about mental health. It will become obvious that each experience is different, and hopefully reflects the framing of work that volunteers have done to try to meet the particular requests and needs of host partners.

The final section relates to the **future of global volunteering**. Chapter 22 presents ideas and hopes for the future of volunteering using **electronic learning possibilities** to enhance existing developments and add innovative ideas for the future of services and learning. Whilst the Covid pandemic has highlighted the gross inequalities of health care around the world, it has also given a boost to the development of digital learning resources and an opportunity to deal with the challenge of climate change by making travel less critical to successful work with international and national colleagues. The final chapter, **global volunteering moving forward**, seeks to contextualise the important considerations raised throughout this book and reflect on the landscape of global volunteering moving forward.

References

1. World Health Organization, 2018. Mental health atlas 2017. Geneva: World Health Organization; 2018. World Health Organization. WHO MiNDbank. www.who.int/mental_health/mindbank/en.

2. Chibanda D, Weiss HA, Verhey R et al. Effect of a primary carebased psychological intervention on symptoms of common mental disorders in Zimbabwe: a randomized clinical trial. JAMA. 2016;316 (24):2618–26. doi:10.1001/jama.2016.19102.

3. World Health Organization. WHO Mental Health Gap Action Programme (mhGAP). 2017. www.who.int/teams/mental-health-and-substance-use/treatment-care/mental-health-gap-action-programme (accessed 1 Jul 2021).

4. World Health Organization. mhGAP Intervention Guide – Version 2.0 for mental, neurological and substance user disorders in non-specialized health settings. 2016. www.who.int/mental_health/mhgap/mhGAP_intervention_guid e_02/en/ (accessed 1 Jul 2021).

5. United Kingdom Foreign Commonwealth and Development Office Travel Advice www.gov.uk/foreign-travel-advice.

6. Haakenstad A, Irvine CMS, Knight M et al. Measuring the availability of human resources for health and its relationship to universal health coverage for 204 countries and territories from 1990 to 2019: a systematic analysis for the Global Burden of Disease Study 2019. The Lancet. 2022.

7. The World Bank. World development indicators: health systems. 2019. Available from: http://wdi.worldbank.org/table/2.12.

8. World Health Organization. Human resources for health – WHO Global Code of Practice on the International Recruitment of Health Personnel: fourth round of national reporting; 2022.

9. Medical Justice. https://medicaljustice.org.uk/volunteering/doctor/.

10. Inter-Agency Standing Committee, 2006. IASC guidelines on mental health and psychosocial support in emergency settings. Geneva, Switzerland: IASC 2006. www.who.int/mental_health/emergen cies/guidelines_iasc_mental_health_psy chosocial_june_2007.pdf (accessed 1 Jul 2021).

11. Sphere Association. The Sphere Handbook: Humanitarian Charter and Minimum Standards in Humanitarian Response, 4th ed. Geneva, Switzerland; 2018. www.spherestandards.org/handbook.

Chapter

1

Background and Principles of Volunteering in Global Mental Health

Peter Hughes and Sam Gnanapragasam

A purposeful, conscientious and well-intentioned mental health volunteer needs to be informed about the background, principles and ethics of global mental health in order to be impactful. This chapter provides background to aid such efforts and introduces global mental health within the wider voluntary context.

Background to Global Mental Health

Mental health is often given low priority or is neglected in health systems worldwide. Although this is true of all settings, including high-income countries, and is dubbed the 'mental health gap', low- and middle-income countries (LMICs) have particular challenges worth noting. The treatment gap between need and access is estimated to be up to 90% in some of the poorest regions in the world[3].

Firstly, owing to the double burden of disease (chronic and communicable diseases), health systems are often stretched. The health burden and financial pressures mean that mental health does not receive adequate funding. Estimates suggest that, on average, spending on mental, neurological and substance use (MNS) disorders is 0.5% in low-income countries and 1.9% in lower- to middle-income countries[5]. Where funded, most of the limited budget for mental health is concentrated in secondary care services with very little community provision for mental health. Often secondary care takes the form of a national hospital, and the service herein may be stretched and standards may be poor, with it catering only for the most ill[6].

Secondly, mental health problems are hugely stigmatised in much of the world. Words for mental illness may be pejorative. People with mental illness are often excluded from active participation in family and community life, and they face discrimination. Research has shown that discrimination often relates to the right to vote (political), the right to inherit property/ make a will (economic), employment (personal) and marriage (personal)[7–10]. Mental illness may be a source of shame and may be believed to have a spiritual underpinning.

Human rights are a core area to consider in global mental health[11]. Those with serious mental illness may be kept at home and even detained there, sometimes in secret. They may be locked in, tied up, chained and treated inhumanely. In doing so, their human rights could be infringed. For those with a disability and other vulnerable groups, there is an increased risk of violations of human rights. Globally in mental health work, health workers are confronted with protection (safeguarding) issues on a regular basis, including domestic/ intimate partner violence, abuse of disabled people and female genital mutilation, to mention just some. One of the important global human rights and laws we need to be aware of is the Convention of the Rights of Persons with Disability (CRPD) which is described below[12].

These challenges are related to funding, as well as stigma and discrimination, and result in those suffering with mental health conditions presenting late to services, or not presenting at all[13,14]. This is particularly the case for vulnerable groups such as women, as there can be increased shame to have female members of the family who are mentally unwell.

For many, the first point of call for any mental health problem is the traditional or spiritual healer[15]. The role they play within communities is varied, but often they contribute to both individual and community identity, as well as helping to shape conceptualisation of wellness and illness. What they do can vary, with some using herbs or religious treatments. There are many traditional healers who work with compassion and diligence and indeed have a deep understanding of local idioms of distress. They may actually complement mental health provision. However, there are others who breach human rights by deprivation of liberty by actions such as beatings, starving and neglect.

Even when people do agree to see a mental health professional, there is usually a severe shortage of these specialists[16]. In many countries, mental health is provided by non-specialists such as general trained doctors, nurses or sometimes laypeople[6]. In some countries, such as Uganda, Ghana and Malawi, there are clinical officers. These are non-doctors, but they are prescribers who provide the backbone of health care in many places where there are no psychiatrists. They are equivalent to the physicians' associates found in the UK. Clinical officers are less likely than doctors to leave their home country, and this means that they are an important cadre to support in global mental health work.

The few trained psychiatrists in LMICs will usually be in the large cities and the chance of consulting a psychiatrist for those people who live rurally or in a village is low. The number of psychiatrists may be further depleted by 'brain drain' where mental health specialists move to other countries or to the private or NGO sector[17]. A further barrier to seeing a psychiatrist is poverty[3]. People often cannot afford to go to see a psychiatrist, travel to a big city (because of the cost of the journey and of lost livelihood) or pay for the medicines prescribed. Medication may be relatively cheap when compared to UK standards, but a long course of treatment can simply be unaffordable for many people.

Even where mental health services are present, there is likely to be varied training standards amongst health staff and poor availability or lack of psychotropic medication. In addition, there may be polypharmacy or limited rational prescribing[18]. People with psychosis can be overmedicated and patients with depression undermedicated, for example. There is a common practice of prescribing vitamins and other medications which may not actually be required. These can be costly for people who cannot afford them.

Overall, the situation for people with mental illness is, sadly, poor in much of the world. This treatment gap is worse in LMICs. However, some of the case examples in this book do show some improvement in mental health across recent years and we can always be optimistic for the future. The principles such as the Sustainable Development Goals (SDGs)[19] described below have put a framework in place and have provided momentum to improve further the situation of people with mental illness in the world. Further, it is important to acknowledge that, given the treatment gap in the UK, even high-income settings are not immune from the challenges and thus we should be open and proactive to any lessons and best practices that can be learnt, adapted and implemented.

International Frameworks in Global Mental Health

This section outlines important international standards, policies, principles and commonly used nomenclature in the field of global mental health. These are essential knowledge for a global volunteer. Although some terms and policies are discussed, this is by no means an exhaustive list. Volunteers are strongly encouraged to do further supplementary reading related to global, regional and local mental health policy and public health principles (see Appendix 1).

Mental Health and Psychosocial Support (MHPSS)

In global mental health and related volunteering, the term *Mental Health and Psychosocial Support* (MHPSS) is currently used rather than mental health. The important underlying principle is to stretch health interventions beyond a narrow medical/pharmacological model and to be able to capture a full range of treatments. It includes the range of support individuals receive to promote their psychosocial well-being and mental state. Support interventions range from individual clinical approaches to those that focus more broadly on financial and social development.

WHO mhGAP Intervention Guide

The WHO mhGAP intervention manual is an excellent guide to some helpful principles of care in managing mental, neurological and substance use (MNS) disorders in a non-specialist setting[20]. It places emphasis on the need for respect, dignity, communication, appropriate assessment and evidenced-based treatment of physical, mental, social and even spiritual domains. This important manual emphasises holistic treatment that incorporates human rights and cultural sensitivity. It can be used by a range of professionals including generalist or primary care doctors, nurses and allied health professionals. The guide provides a series of algorithms to aid clinical decision-making. It is available for free across online formats, as well as on mobile devices through an app.

The Sustainable Development Goals (SDGs) 2013–2030

These are UN internationally agreed goals launched in 2015, with the aim to achieve them by 2030[19, 21]. Goal number three is on health. This goal is to ensure healthy lives and to promote well-being across the whole age spectrum. There are particular targets on suicide and substance use. There are 16 other goals including environmental sustainability, poverty, education, gender equality, peace and justice, all of which interrelate with health. As a volunteer it is worth remembering these different areas. Mental health is a complex area with multifactorial aetiology and management plans. Climate, water supply, conflict and gender inequality all have effects on the genesis of mental health problems. Health, poverty and injustice all go hand in hand.

WHO World Mental Health Action Plan 2013–2020

The WHO World Mental Health Action Plan 2013–2020[22], now extended to 2030, is another useful background guidance for volunteers. It has four main principles:

o Good governance and leadership
o Community-based services
o Prevention and promotion strategies
o Good information technology

These four principles are useful reference points when volunteers ask the question, 'what can I do?'. A volunteer can find themselves doing things they weren't expecting, such as supporting leadership skills, the promotion of mental health and record keeping, as well as training specifically in mental health.

Inter-Agency Standing Committee (IASC): Principles of Humanitarian Responses

In humanitarian settings there are principles enshrined in the Inter-Agency Standing Committee (IASC) Guidelines on Mental Health and Psychosocial Support (MHPSS) in Emergency Settings[23]. This committee of experts on humanitarian emergencies devised principles for responding in these situations. An important element of this is not to work in isolation but alongside others to ensure that no harm is done, and that there is a co-ordinated benefit. There are many areas of specific guidance that should be followed in humanitarian settings. For example, IASC outlines how to support psychiatric hospitals after emergencies.

Convention of the Rights of Persons with Disability (CRPD)

This important United Nations convention from 2006 to 2008 is hugely influential on the human rights of people with disabilities. The convention includes mental illness as a disability. According to CRPD[12], people with mental illness or psychosocial disability (the preferred term used) should be empowered to be fully participating members of society with access to health, education, justice and family life, etc. It fits with the recovery model of mental illness. Although ratified in many countries, it is patchily implemented in most of the world. It has important implications in how we conduct our psychiatry services.

Mental Health Law and Legislation

Mental health laws, where present, protect the rights of people with mental illness/psycho-social disability. This is particularly relevant for people who are in psychiatric hospitals. It is important to recognise that many countries have no mental health laws or have ones that often date from colonial and/or historic times. Volunteers need to be aware of the laws of the country they visit.

Background to Volunteering

The Oxford Dictionary definition of a volunteer is 'a person who freely offers to take part in an enterprise or undertake a task'[24]. Global volunteering in mental health aims to utilise available skills and resources to improve the well-being and mental health of all people from all countries, religions, genders, ages, cultures, socio-economic backgrounds, sexual orientation, beliefs and disabilities. Volunteering in global mental health is responsive to local need rather than directed by UK volunteers. It is usually mutually beneficial.

As volunteers, it is necessary to appreciate, consider and reflect on the contemporary and historical socio-economic, political and cultural context in which volunteering is undertaken. This is particularly important as volunteers from the UK. On one hand, the UK has a long history of volunteering in other countries around the world and there is value in volunteering by trained specialists from the UK. This individual voluntary spirit has been supported by wider governmental priorities – for example, the UK was one of the few countries to commit to 0.7% of GDP for overseas development up to 2021 (note it is now 0.5%). On the other hand, the complex colonial history of the UK and the perceptions of the empire in the recipient countries cannot be ignored. This can still be, understandably, a shadow over work that UK volunteers do globally. Indeed, it is also important to recognise the ongoing systemic causes of inequity that prevailing economic and geo-political factors contribute to in relation to trade, migration and climate challenges.

In his 2007 report Lord Crisp, demonstrated the value of UK volunteering globally and highlighted the value of UK health professionals volunteering in other countries and how this could produce mutual benefit. This report was a spur to some of the current volunteering. The UK parliament produced an All-Party Volunteering Report similarly valuing global health work[25]. The UK commitment to volunteering is exemplified by the Global Health Exchange and UK Med. Health Education England supports Global Health Exchange which provides volunteering opportunities for all professions in the NHS in England to work globally for mutual benefit. UK Med was set up by the UK government to focus humanitarian health expertise in cases of disasters.

There are a number of similar examples of health volunteering across the other regions of Wales, Scotland and Northern Ireland. It is important to be able to justify volunteering globally whilst there are needs at home in the UK, including prevailing inequalities. However, this is not mutually exclusive. Chapter 5 in this book outlines how global volunteering helps the health system of origin (e.g. NHS services) as well as our partner host countries through higher-skilled health, with more satisfied workers returning.

There is a long history of UK psychiatrists volunteering overseas from the NHS, diaspora groups and others. They have helped make significant and sustainable contributions in those countries. The roles of such volunteers have also included organisations such as the United Nations (UN), international non-governmental organisations (INGOs) and other organisations, as well as individually.

This book recognises the limits of volunteering and the geo-political, economic and historical structures that continue to perpetuate inequality around the world. Nonetheless, we highlight the positive impact that volunteers can make to address this gap even a little and aid the movement towards a more just world. In doing so, we accept and advocate for the need to move beyond aid and the voluntary model to a justice and rights-based model in international health governance.

Case Study: The Royal College of Psychiatry Volunteering Project[1]

The Royal College of Psychiatrists (RCPsych) set up a volunteer programme to support work in global mental health. It began with Professor Andrew Sims as president of the College in 2002, in response to the paucity of psychiatrists globally. His aim was to provide a link between UK psychiatric expertise and needs identified by partners globally. As a college with many international medical graduates and international divisions, developing volunteering was important for a global college. The College has been supporting global volunteering since the formation of the volunteer scheme. Subsequent presidents continued this support, particularly Sheila Hollins during her presidential term. She organised a fundraising trek and championed awareness of the value of volunteering.

The programme works through the College holding a list of registered psychiatry volunteers who are then matched with requests from hosts overseas. This means that the College stamp is on these assignments and there is oversight on the quality of the work and good governance. Many NGOs and other organisations request at least six months duration for any volunteering. Pragmatically, this scheme has a focus on shorter-term international trips, between several weeks to three-month assignments. This is because this is generally the maximum time psychiatrists can be released from their employment. There have been upwards of 60 assignments since the scheme started. Some of these are described more fully in this book. The Sudan volunteering programme is one example of making the most of short-term assignments by arranging for a series of overlapping volunteer psychiatrists to be integrated into a local postgraduate course for primary care doctors[2]. The teaching was co-facilitated by both the UK psychiatrists and Sudanese psychiatrists and psychologists after an initial trainers' workshop. It is described in Chapter 21. This was a partnership between the RCPsych, WHO, Ministry of Health and a local university. Online supervision followed the face-to-face stage.

Similarly, for Myanmar and Kashmir there have been imaginative ways of making the most of the limited time of individual volunteers, which have helped to make the projects more longer-term. This is described in Chapters 13 and 20, respectively. There is a new Royal College of Psychiatrists' International Strategy (2020)[4] with a plan to scale up volunteering to about 100 volunteer activities per year. This includes opportunities to develop new volunteering projects.

Effect of the Covid-19 Pandemic

The Covid-19 pandemic has shown the potential to work and collaborate virtually without the need for travel. This technological catalyst in virtual working allows volunteers to respect the climate in avoiding unnecessary flight travel. Some very recent examples of successful electronic voluntary work during lockdown have been delivering a whole mental health course (mhGAP) online to health workers in Gaza, giving subspecialty lectures in north-west Syria and supporting the academic programme of psychiatry trainees in Bethlehem. The Royal College of Psychiatrists has also delivered global webinars. Volunteers are continuing to provide online supervision to health workers throughout the world.

At the same time, the pandemic has also shown us the limits of virtual working and the benefits of on-the-ground presence and collaboration. It remains to be fully evaluated how efficacious these online partnerships prove to be, compared to face-to-face working. It is clear that there is a preference for face-to-face work when possible. So much of global volunteering is about building networks and understanding the local environment which can only be done face to face. On a practical level the internet connectivity of much of the world poses a big challenge to online volunteering. However, it is likely that future volunteering, overall, will involve some form of hybrid online and face-to-face volunteering.

Principles of Volunteering in Global Mental Health

The important principles that direct the focus of any intervention in volunteering are described below. It is about people. It is about investing in people, including oneself[26].

Do No Harm

One of the key principles that is embedded in volunteering is the maxim of doing no harm. *Primum non nocere*: first do no harm – this is a very old phrase constantly repeated to every generation of clinicians. This must be the top principle. A volunteer needs to work in a professionalised, ethical and evidence-based way. Sometimes the harm that can be done is not immediately apparent. There is a need to always listen to advice to ensure that our interventions are helpful and cause no direct or indirect harm.

Examples of harmful practices:
- Training without follow-up supervision is an example of potentially doing harm as knowledge and skills can get corrupted
- Training people inadequately may lead to faulty practice without adequate supervision
- Telling people what to do or saying they have wrong ideas or behaviour is usually counterproductive
- Abuse of drugs or alcohol in public
- When too much focus is placed on trauma at the expense of supporting people through common and complex mental health problems and building on strength
- Having a special or research interest and using a host population for this may do harm and is probably unethical. For example, diagnosis of post-traumatic stress disorder can be casual at times and overdiagnosed

Justice and Solidarity, Not Charity

Justice for all is a key ideal. Justice is an important part of well-being[11]. It is not always possible to change things ourselves. Volunteers need to be informed and not appear naïve and listen to the stories being told. It is one of the difficulties of volunteering that they can often feel powerless as they hear terrible stories of injustice. They can listen but must never collude with injustice. They need advice on anything else they can do. This emphasises the importance of good supervision and mentoring for any volunteer. There is a movement in global volunteering to speak out against injustices. The remit of the organisation MSF (Medécins Sans Frontières/Doctors without Borders) is just that. They bear testament to injustice. In reality, what can be said can be more nuanced for the risk of causing harm to any project. Volunteers can be removed from a project and country. The project can be shut down. It takes experience, maturity and good advice on how to deal with injustices.

Attention needs to be given to any outdated ideas of 'white saviour' or 'neo-imperialistic altruism'. Modern volunteering is about partnership, solidarity and justice, and not charity.

Human Rights

It cannot be overstated that it is very important to respect human rights as core principles in volunteering[27]. If there are violations of human rights it is necessary to speak about this in an appropriate way. This is where supervision can be important to help frame this. It is important to respect culture without accepting things that can be called cultural but are fundamentally violating human rights, such as domestic violence and female genital mutilation (FGM).

In countries where there are obvious or gross violations of human rights, it can be an ethical challenge to decide whether it is better to stay away or to go and try to help build better services for people with mental illness. There may be increased risks to training programmes, as well as personal safety, if violations are challenged. It is worth taking advice and working with organisations that are accustomed to dealing with this. It is inappropriate and unprofessional to give a lecture to people on what is wrong with their country or the way they work.

Evidence-Based Practice

It is important to be able to justify interventions in LMICs. It is clear in the past that there was little research or formal evaluation of health interventions within such contexts[28]. For example, while 85% of the global population live in LMICs, only 6% of mental health published literature in indexed journals used to come from such settings.

This is now changing, and there is a growing wealth of research on global health interventions.

Important literature to read includes the Lancet Commission on Global Mental Health and Sustainable Development in 2007 and then in 2018. This showed that mental health can be treated effectively in LMICs. The cost-effectiveness of treating mental illness is now proven. Non-specialists can be trained to deliver effective mental health care. This research underpins the important principle of integrated mental health in primary care, using trained non-specialist health workers.

As such, there is an obligation on volunteers to utilise and implement evidence-based measures. When deviating from this, stringent monitoring and evaluation is a requirement of any project from the very beginning, and metrics should be co-produced with local service providers and users where possible.

It is to be noted that while programmatic evaluation does not require ethical approval, any research studies or undertakings will need this. This can take some time to get, particularly when both UK and host country ethical approval may be needed. As such, research volunteers would benefit immensely, and indeed would be ethnically obliged to co-develop such research projects with local researchers and clinicians, including where it pertains to project ownership and authorship.

Recognition of Competency, and Limits

In the UK there is a regulated high standard of training for professionals in health and social services. Volunteers can feel confident in their training and how this can be of value to others. However, despite the level of training, it is important to recognise that the training often relates to the UK context and may have significant shortcomings when seeking to be applied elsewhere. Similarly, those without formal training in a UK context will likely have a richer understanding of the local contributors and idioms of distress.

Professional Standing

A volunteer who has come through an organisation such as the Royal College of Psychiatrists bears an important brand and identity that carries a huge impact in many parts of the world. This helps to be confident about the quality of training and skills that can be shared with the world, as well as building up knowledge and experiences from volunteering globally. Legally, it may be necessary to be professionally registered in the country one volunteers in, particularly if one is doing any clinical work. It is essential to follow the law of the country in which one is volunteering.

There are currently no legislative rules for volunteering. However, the volunteering must be professional and, for psychiatrists, match the Royal College of Psychiatrists' values of courage, innovation, respect, collaboration, learning and excellence, as well as abiding by General Medical Council standards. Other professions should espouse their organisational standards. The volunteer is likely to need to register with the local regulatory authority. Volunteering programmes will have accountability and professionalism structures built in.

Capacity Building, Sustainable Volunteering, Human Resources

Volunteering should never be done in isolation. It is important for the volunteer to fit in with the national principles and policies of health service and to be well-informed about the country they are invited to visit, this is discussed in Chapter 6 entitled Preparation. Where possible, volunteers should be conducting training and building capacity more than doing clinical work. If there is a need for clinical work, then this should always be seen as a training opportunity for local health workers. Volunteers should not be a substitution for missing clinicians but should work to strengthen the capacity of existing health workers. Examples that have been helpful, apart from the usual general training, include training in rapid tranquillisation principles and breakaway technique.

Global volunteering is almost always an exercise in supporting human resource and system capacity. The term capacity building is often used in developmental and voluntary circles to describe this. Your role as part of capacity building is often in helping to make an investment in the existing health system and the health workers, to allow them to be more capable of managing patients' care. This is through training and building up skills. Another term used is 'task shifting'. This means that health workers, who may not have had the years of mental health training as a specialist psychiatrist, are tasked with service delivery of specific tasks through specific training[29].

Long-Term Commitments

The ideal is to commit to a longer period as a volunteer. Usually there is a six-month minimum period for many organisations. There are many different schemes that have shown long-term commitment over years with a regular supply of volunteers such as the Scottish Malawi project[30] or King's Somaliland/Sierra Leone partnership[31]. One of the highlights described by one volunteer is delivering face-to-face training and following up within two days through an online portal with the very same participants. The Sudan project described in this book in Chapter 19 is an example of a project where short-term volunteering led to a longer more sustainable partnership project[2]. There was a succession of volunteers from around the world who co-ordinated efforts to produce more sustainable useful training followed by online supervision.

Recognition of Vulnerable Groups Such as Women and Children

Women and children are the most vulnerable, generally, in LMICs. An important principle is to gear any programme around their needs. In LMICs, families are very important, and the mother is the linchpin of the community. Women are reported to have higher rates of many mental health conditions. Women are particularly at risk from poverty, poor nutrition and bad housing. They need support to obtain their rights. Children depend on their mothers' good mental health to develop themselves. In some countries women are not able to consent to their own medical procedures. For example, in some countries in the African continent, a woman must have consent from her husband to have a caesarean section. In other places, women can be prevented by their families from seeing doctors. Seeing a male doctor or health worker may be unacceptable to them even if it is at the cost of the woman's health. For all these reasons care for women is crucial. Once a woman's mental health is improved, the whole family and the community will benefit.

Culture

As mentioned throughout this book, attention to and appreciation of culture is essential[32]. All volunteers need to make every effort to be fully briefed on the culture of where they go. Volunteers need to respect local values and customs. Even for diaspora volunteers, they may need to remember that their home country has changed. Paradoxically, sometimes diaspora volunteers may be seen as outsiders. There can be a very complex dynamic as we see in Chapter 16.

The UK volunteer will do well to try to understand what the local traditional healers are doing through having respectful and inquisitive conversations with local stakeholders. If there is abuse, this is a serious ethical issue. The volunteer needs to broach this sensitively with their hosts and their UK-based supervisor. The answer to this issue needs to come from the host community.

Supervision and Professional Development

A volunteer needs to be self-reflective and informed. A volunteer needs to engage in continuous professional development, be regularly supervised and evaluated as well as reflecting with peers on their practice, in the way normally expected of UK practitioners.

Day-to-Day Pace, and Flexibility

It takes years to change services and embed new training into regular practice. Volunteers usually need to slow down from the pace of working in their home countries. A volunteer may be starting, or being part of the start, of an ongoing long-term process. Returning home is often when volunteers realise what a frantic pace they work at back home and this can be a learning point for their own well-being.

Flexibility and attention must be applied to individual and host needs. Every volunteering assignment is different, which is why it can be such an exciting opportunity. Any volunteer needs to be flexible and, in a sense, be a doctor, nurse, psychologist and social worker, as well as possessing other management, leadership and logistical skills. Volunteers often have to mobilise skills in education, well-being, livelihood (employment) as well as other areas that map on to the sustainable development goals (SDGs). This recognition and application is not only valuable during the voluntary placement, but it also makes doctors, nurses, psychologists and social workers better at their work upon return to the country of origin as it broadens and accelerates professional skill development.

Psychological Adaptation of the Volunteer Role

Personal adaptation is an important underlying principle in volunteers, and this is often varied depending on the timescale of the assignment. Even for shorter term international work, personal adjustment is an important principle. Whilst this varies from person to person, for many there are different stages. For example, with a 12-week assignment, week one to two is often said to be characterised by a sense of panic and questioning of role, and it may be accompanied by feeling overwhelmed. Weeks four to eight is often the period of settling into the local community. Weeks eight to twelve may be intense due to the pressure to complete the stated objectives and ensure the sustainability of programmatic work. The next phase is returning home and adjusting. For some, it is an addictive process and there will be an urge to repeat global volunteering. For others, there is satisfaction and a return to normal 'civilian' life. In almost all stages outlined, most feel a deep sense of purpose and fulfilment.

Learning from Mistakes

Mistakes are natural in everyday life and in clinical medicine. It is important to be mindful of this and to make every effort to learn from mistakes that we make during the course of volunteering. Further, it is useful to reflect on the mistakes commonly made by volunteers and learn from this:

- Having a donor mentality and not one of partnership
- Doing clinical work rather than more sustainable activities such as training
- Not being prepared for the host/voluntary context before departure
- Overestimating, or underestimating, baseline knowledge and skills of local health workers
- Getting over-involved and not keeping professional and personal boundaries
- Doing harm. This remains the most troubling possibility.

Table 1.1 Do's of volunteering

Do's of volunteering
- Do no harm
- Do slow down and then slow down again
- Learn
- Develop partnerships
- Be flexible
- Prepare
- Follow guidelines
- Learn what are affordable, available drugs
- Show humility
- Respect culture
- Follow human rights
- Look after yourself
- Bring enough money to manage
- Follow FCDO guidelines
- Keep well with vaccinations/yellow card
- Wear seat belt

Table 1.2 Don'ts of volunteering

Don'ts of volunteering
- Volunteer in isolation
- Be UK/country of origin centric
- 'Try to save the world' – it takes years to make changes
- Do not give money away – you have to say 'no' to requests
- Support pharmaceutical companies prescribing teaching without emphasis on evidence based practice and decision making
- Substitute services that will disappear when you leave

Conclusion

It is important to embark on any volunteering well-prepared with knowledge of the relevant background and principles. This should also be the basis of all future volunteering projects. What is important is the professionalisation of volunteering. A volunteer needs to be following the same standards of professional work as in their home country. A volunteer also needs to be mindful of the ethical issues and be aware of their own lack of knowledge of facts on the ground and how to skilfully negotiate through difficult and sensitive areas. It is important to understand the nature of the treatment gap that exists around the world, and the challenges mental health services face in the context of the competing large burden of disease. There are also challenges related to stigma and human rights, as these often result in delays in accessing care. A range of international frameworks offer guidance, and these include the WHO mhGAP Intervention Guide, SDGs, IASC guidelines and the Global Mental Health Action Plan 2013–2030. Volunteering must first do no harm, and then seek to build upon acts of justice and solidarity in an attempt to build sustainable, evidence-based and culturally appropriate systems.

References

1. Royal College of Psychiatrists. Global volunteering scheme of the Royal College of Psychiatrists.

2. Ali S, Saeed K, Hughes P. Evaluation of a mental health training project in the republic of the Sudan using the mental health gap action programme curriculum. International Psychiatry. 2012;9(2):43–5.

3. Patel V, Maj M, Flisher AJ et al. Reducing the treatment gap for mental disorders: a WPA survey. World Psychiatry. 2010;9 (3):169–76.

4. Royal College of Psychiatrists. International strategy 2020. www .rcpsych.ac.uk/docs/default-source/mem bers/international-divisions/rcpsych-international-strategy.pdf.

5. Jacob K, Sharan P, Mirza I et al. Mental health systems in countries: where are we now? The Lancet. 2007;370(9592):1061–77.

6. Patel V, Minas H, Cohen A et al. Global Mental Health: Principles and Practice. Oxford University Press; 2013.

7. Bhugra D. Social Discrimination and Social Justice. Taylor & Francis; 2016. pp. 336–41.

8. Bhugra D, Pathare S, Gosavi C et al. Mental illness and the right to vote: a review of legislation across the world. International Review of Psychiatry. 2016;28(4):395–9.

9. Bhugra D, Pathare S, Nardodkar R et al. Legislative provisions related to marriage and divorce of persons with mental health problems: a global review. International Review of Psychiatry. 2016;28(4):386–92.

10. Bhugra D, Pathare S, Joshi R et al. Right to property, inheritance, and contract and persons with mental illness. International Review of Psychiatry. 2016;28(4):402–8.

11. Slim H. Humanitarian Action and Ethics. Bloomsbury Publishing; 2018.

12. United Nations. Convention on the Rights of Persons with Disabilities; 2013.

13. Hughes P. Psychiatry in Sudan: a personal experience. Psychiatric Bulletin. 1996;20(1):46–7.

14. Zolezzi M, Alamri M, Shaar S et al. Stigma associated with mental illness and its treatment in the Arab culture: a systematic review. International Journal of Social Psychiatry. 2018;64(6):597–609.

15. Nortje G, Oladeji B, Gureje O et al. Effectiveness of traditional healers in treating mental disorders: a systematic review. The Lancet Psychiatry. 2016;3(2):154–70.

16. World Health Organization. Mental health atlas 2017 Geneva: World Health Organization; 2018. https://apps.who.int/iris/handle/10665/272735.

17. Gureje O, Hollins S, Botbol M et al. Report of the WPA task force on brain drain. World Psychiatry. 2009;8(2):115.

18. Morrato EH, Dodd S, Oderda G et al. Prevalence, utilization patterns, and predictors of antipsychotic polypharmacy: experience in a multistate Medicaid population, 1998–2003. Clinical Therapeutics. 2007;29(1):183–95.

19. United Nations. Transforming our world: the 2030 Agenda for Sustainable Development. UN General Assembly; 2015.

20. World Health Organization. mhGAP intervention guide for mental, neurological and substance use disorders in non-specialized health settings: mental health Gap Action Programme (mhGAP). World Health Organization; 2016.

21. Votruba N, Thornicroft G, Group FS. Sustainable development goals and mental health: learnings from the contribution of the FundaMentalSDG global initiative. Global Mental Health. 2016;3.

22. World Health Organization. Mental health action plan 2013–2020. Geneva: World Health Organization; 2013.

23. Committee I-AS. IASC guidelines on mental health and psychosocial support in emergency settings. Geneva, Switzerland: IASC; 2006.

24. Oxford Dictionary of English. Oxford University Press; 2021.

25. All-Party Parliamentary Group on Mental Health and All-Party Parliamentary Group on Global Health. Mental Health for Sustainable Development. London: All-Party Parliamentary Group on Mental Health; 2014.

26. Hughes P. UK mental health professionals volunteering in LMIC – benefits to UK and host countries; 2015.

27. Assembly UG. Universal declaration of human rights. UN General Assembly. 1948;302(2):14–25.

28. Saxena S, Paraje G, Sharan P et al. The 10/90 divide in mental health research: trends over a 10-year period. The British Journal of Psychiatry. 2006;188(1):81–2.

29. Patel V. The future of psychiatry in low-and middle-income countries. Psychological Medicine. 2009;39(11):1759–62.

30. Scotland-Malawi Mental Health Education Project. Malawi quick guide to mental health. SMMHEP.

31. King's College London CfGHHP. King's Global Health Partnerships.

32. Bhugra D, Craig T, Bhui K. Mental Health of Refugees and Asylum Seekers. Oxford University Press; 2010.

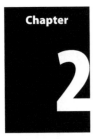

Humanitarian Emergencies

Peter Hughes

Introduction

Whenever there is a humanitarian emergency in the world, mental health workers in the UK and other regions may wish to offer their skills. For diaspora health workers it may be an even more agonising longing as they see news footage from their childhood and familial homes. However, unless the volunteer follows proper internationally accepted guidelines there is a risk that that same health worker will end up not just being unhelpful but becoming a burden on the relief effort. This chapter considers volunteering in humanitarian emergencies and related principles, and includes some personal reflections.

Background

The terms 'humanitarian crisis' and 'humanitarian emergency' are used interchangeably to mean 'an event or series of events that represents a critical threat to the health, safety, security or wellbeing of a community or other large group of people, usually over a wide area'[1]. Such events may be man-made crises such as armed conflicts, natural disasters such as earthquakes, or may be complex emergencies (a combination of both man-made and natural disasters).

The number of humanitarian emergencies varies per year. Climate change is likely to lead to more emergencies in the future and a chronic ecological crisis[2]. For example, in Bangladesh there are already annual cyclones and due to sea-level related changes, they are likely to be a major victim of climate change. It is undoubtedly true that the lower income countries of the world face the brunt of these natural disasters, wars and other disasters[3].

In 2020, the world faced an unprecedented emergency with the Covid-19 pandemic. This has been unparalleled in its range of effects and has taken spontaneous local volunteering to our doorsteps. There are other emergencies that have become chronic situations, such as that of refugees. As of 2022, there are around 27 million refugees in the world now according to UNHCR. Humanitarian emergencies expose weak health systems. Health care can break down quickly. Health is one of the biggest basic needs after a disaster, with increased demand at a time when services are most depleted[4]. Emergency responses need to be fast and flexible to meet changing needs. Governments may struggle to work at the required pace of the emergency response. There can be unexpected hurdles. At the same time, sometimes in emergencies, the bureaucracy and red tape may be removed[5].

When the emergency phase is over then things may slow down. They may slow down too much, and it may be very frustrating facing urgent needs and knowing, for example, that essential materials needed are locked up in a port warehouse. Items such as medication, mosquito nets and water purifying kits can be held up whilst logistics get sorted.

Humanitarian response works by building on the strengths of what is working well already (or has potential), engaging key people and mitigating the negative aspects such as violence, corruption and opportunistic exploitation[6].

Types of Problems and Prevalence

In any emergency situation, there are a range of social and mental health challenges. Emergencies impact an individual by limiting the ability to function and cope with everyday tasks in life, and they also strip away the infrastructure, people and systems that usually serve them and their loved ones[7]. The WHO helpfully prompts consideration of some of these challenges, summarised in Table 2.1.

In emergency situations, most individuals express some distress. This may be characterised by feelings of sadness, anxiety, hopelessness, irritability or anger. They may also have physical manifestations through symptoms of fatigue, pain and generalised aches. This is normal and, in time, such symptoms will improve. They are often transient reactions to loss. For some, however, symptoms remain and meet the threshold of a mental health disorder. They become chronic and will eventually impact the day-to-day functioning of both the individual and related communities. This is a key difference that must be recognised during a humanitarian crisis – distinguishing emotional distress from mental health disorder[9]. In addition to these groups of individuals, there are others with pre-existing mental health conditions in whom an emergency causes significant vulnerability. This may be due to loss of support systems, as well as access to medication and/or health services. In addition to this, they may be differentially impacted by the stressors related to the emergency and thus may experience an exacerbation of symptoms, or even a relapse.

Estimates of mental health disorder vary due to different contexts, the nature of the emergencies and the study methodology. A meta-analysis that pooled some of these studies in conflict settings found a point prevalence of mental disorders (depression, anxiety, post-traumatic stress disorder, bipolar disorder and schizophrenia) of 22.1%[10]. It is thought that pre-existing mental health conditions can relapse following humanitarian emergencies and overall rates double in frequency. As a psychiatrist you may need to see or support the treatment of clinical cases, and these may be complex.

It is also important to recognise that some people retain good mental health, and this is owing to a range of individual and societal support. They may even experience post-traumatic growth.

Table2.1 Examples of social and mental health problems in emergencies[8]

	Social problems	Mental health problems
Pre-existing	Poverty and discrimination of marginalised groups	Mental disorders such as depression, schizophrenia or harmful use of alcohol
Emergency-induced	Family separation, lack of safety, loss of livelihoods, disrupted social networks and low trust and resources	Grief, acute stress reactions, harmful use of alcohol and drugs and depression and anxiety, including post-traumatic stress disorder
Humanitarian response-induced	Overcrowding, lack of privacy and undermining of community or traditional support	Anxiety due to a lack of information about food distribution or about how to obtain basic services

Principles

This section outlines the principles of humanitarian emergency response:

1. **Preparedness**: Each country should have a preparedness plan for any disaster[4]. For example, Bangladesh, which is very prone to natural disasters, has plans for the inevitable yearly cyclones. There can be practice runs for responding to disasters.

2. The response in any case will be **multisectoral,** involving military, health, education, nutrition, logistic, livelihood and myriad other areas[4,11]. Countries, ideally, can manage their own disaster response but can easily be overwhelmed. This is usually in low-resource countries but even in the HICs, services can be overwhelmed; for example, the 2005 Hurricane Katrina in Louisiana, USA.

3. A principle that is useful to follow is **'building back better'**[12]. A disaster may be an opportunity for long-term sustainable development. The WHO has produced a document of this same name highlighting case studies of disasters where long-term sustainable improvement followed an emergency. A good example is Sri Lanka after the tsunami of 2004. The service developed after the disaster led to a much better, more accessible community-based mental health care system.

4. A key principle is **co-ordination** and this is important for the volunteer to understand [4]. Never work in isolation. In humanitarian settings, individuals can be seen operating out of great goodwill to help their home country but not effectively, as it is not possible to make a constructive impact without co-ordination with national partners.

5. Response to a humanitarian emergency needs to include all elements quite rapidly. There is some order, however. For the international volunteer, first there is the need to assure that their **own safety and needs** are met.

6. There is a need for a **situation or needs analysis** to identify needs and priorities. For example, there may be a hugely increased need for health care, shelter, nutrition and security. The 4Ws is a mapping exercise which looks at Who is doing What, Where and When[13]. This will tell you where you fit in and not duplicate what others are doing.

Steps in a humanitarian response by following Inter-Agency Standing Committee (IASC) guidelines[4]

- Review of all available information and learning from other similar disasters
- Ensure that response is locally led
- Situation analysis – needs assessment
- Co-ordination group led by host country
- Respond to basic needs and security
- 4Ws – mapping exercise: Who is doing What, Where and When
- Monitoring and evaluation systems
- Medication supply – psychotropic
- Support human resources
- Strengthen existing structures and community supports
- Provide good reliable information on disaster and resources available
- Training and capacity building

A volunteer can be a very useful support to local leaders and even government representatives. Charities like Médecins Sans Frontières (MSF) and International Medical Corps (IMC) are some of the excellent organisations with which one can volunteer in humanitarian emergencies. A volunteer can fit in well in organisations such as these and be very useful. What is not helpful is individuals travelling independently, even when part of the diaspora, and not following the principles of emergency response. Examples of bad practice are standalone surveys or mental health silo clinics that are not part of co-ordinated work and thus not sustainable.

Tools for Working in Humanitarian Settings

Some of the useful tools we can use in emergencies are psychological first aid (PFA)[14] and WHO mhGAP Humanitarian version[15]. It is helpful to be familiar and proficient in these tools even before deployment to an emergency situation.

Psychological First Aid

Psychological first aid (PFA) is a non-specialist approach to dealing with people in distress in humanitarian emergencies. One of the tasks in humanitarian emergencies is to train and implement PFA amongst first responders. This can be health workers, ambulance drivers, even grave diggers and burial teams.

The principles of PFA are about meeting basic needs, including accurate information and supportive, humane and practical help. In practice this means making sure people have shelter, food to eat and a phone to use to contact family. Practical examples include providing money for bus fare or telephone access for those affected to reconnect with their family. This is simple, basic practical help which can mean so much in emergency settings. When people are overwhelmed and PFA is not sufficient then they need to be referred to more formal health services.

mhGAP Humanitarian InterventionGuide

The other useful tool is the WHO mhGAP Humanitarian version[15]. This is a shorter manual than the mhGAP InterventionGuide and focuses on conditions that are more prominent in humanitarian emergencies.

Inter-Agency Standing Committee (IASC) and SPHERE Guidelines

This guide covers all levels of health services from the specialised, primary care, community to basic services/security. Each area will have needs identified that can be looked at. There can be no health without basic needs and security being met. Mental health should be accessible at primary health care level. It is important to support community assistance, for example community leaders. Specialist services may be neglected and need support with basic needs, medication and staffing. Co-ordination is key with all stakeholders. An important principle of these guidelines is 'do no harm'. There are many other aspects which need to be followed in emergency settings.

Reflections

Personal reflections can be found in the humanitarian field narratives in Chapter 18. Here, there is greater focus with specific examples of work in Chad, Darfur, Haiti, Sierra Leone and Bangladesh, respectively. Themes considered include self-care, clinical volunteering and non-clinical volunteering in the context of humanitarian settings.

Conclusion

Humanitarian emergencies pose a critical threat to the safety, security and well-being of the communities affected. These emergencies are devastating for local populations and are likely to be evergrowing with the climate crisis. As volunteers, there is the potential to support local populations. To do this, it is necessary to adhere to key humanitarian response principles. These include a deep acknowledgement of cultural issues and the dynamic of outside help in a host country. If applied well, humanitarian work is truly transformative for the volunteer. The memories never go away. Sometimes it can be dramatic like on television, but much of it is training in a hall, open air or office and sitting in meetings. It is important to always be professional and follow the guidelines. You, as a volunteer, can make a difference.

References

1. Humanitarian Coalition. What is a Humanitarian Emergency? 2022. www .humanitariancoalition.ca/what-is-a-huma nitarian-emergency.

2. Wahlström M. Before the next disaster strikes – the humanitarian impact of climate change. UN Chronicle online edition; 2007.

3. Walker P, Glasser J, Kambli S. Climate change as a driver of humanitarian crises and response. Feinstein International Center; 2012.

4. Inter-Agency Standing Committee IASC guidelines on mental health and psychosocial support in emergency settings. Geneva, Switzerland: IASC 2006; 2006.

5. Rose N, Hughes P, Ali S et al. Integrating mental health into primary health care settings after an emergency: lessons from Haiti. Intervention. 2011;9(3):211–24.

6. Slim H. Humanitarian Action and Ethics. Bloomsbury Publishing; 2018.

7. Colliard C, Bizouerne C, Corna F et al. The psychosocial impact of humanitarian crises: a better understanding for better interventions. ACF-International [Google Scholar]; 2014.

8. World Health Organization. Fact Sheet: Mental health in emergencies; 2019. www .who.int/news-room/fact-sheets/detail/me ntal-health-in-emergencies.

9. Horwitz AV. Distinguishing distress from disorder as psychological outcomes of stressful social arrangements. Health. 2007;11(3):273–89.

10. Charlson F, van Ommeren M, Flaxman A et al. New WHO prevalence estimates of mental disorders in conflict settings: a systematic review and meta-analysis. The Lancet. 2019;394(10194):240–8.

11. Sphere Association. Sphere handbook: Humanitarian Charter and Minimum Standards in Humanitarian Response. Practical Action; 2018.

12. World Health Organization. Building back better: sustainable mental health care after emergencies. World Health Organization; 2013.

13. IASC Reference Group for Mental Health and Psychosocial Support in Emergency Settings. Who is Where, When, doing What (4Ws) in Mental Health and Psychosocial Support; 2012.

14. World Health Organization. Psychological First Aid: Guide for Field Workers. World Health Organization; 2011.

15. World Health Organization. mhGAP Humanitarian Intervention Guide

(mhGAP-HIG): clinical management of mental, neurological and substance use conditions in humanitarian emergencies. World Health Organization; 2015.

16. Brooks S, Amlot R, Rubin GJ et al. Psychological resilience and post-traumatic growth in disaster-exposed organisations: overview of the literature. BMJ Mil Health. 2020;166(1):52–6.

17. Hughes P. Mental illness and health in Sierra Leone affected by Ebola: lessons for health workers. Intervention. 2015;13(1):60–9.

Ethical Issues in Global Volunteering: An Ethicist's Perspective

Ayesha Ahmad

Introduction

Travelling with the purpose of volunteering in mental health involves recognising and responding to those who are suffering. The motivations for such global movements in mental health are clear when considering the moral sense of justice, rights and values that form the backbone of medicine's history and practice. However, psychiatry presents us with complex particularities that challenge our ethical reflection of global volunteering in mental health. This chapter explores the ways that the fundamental principles of medical ethics and dilemmas from the perspective of a western-trained volunteer are embroiled and embedded in the concepts of the mind, self, suffering and surrounding worlds.

Overview

Ethical principles are fundamental underlying tenets of all clinical practice; every encounter with another individual is essentially an ethical encounter. Yet, ethical issues tend to be discussed only when there are conflicts or dilemmas or problems. When clinical practice enters the humanitarian or global sphere, ethics is often extrapolated in terms of cultural clashes and reduced to singular experiences, rather than conceptualising the event of humanitarianism and its meaning for a particular context. Such an oversight is even more paramount in a time whereby volunteering in humanitarian settings can be a matter of popularism and coincides with the parallel movement of global mental health. This chapter formulates key ethical principles of volunteering in humanitarian psychiatry. There is a call to develop a more robust phenomenological inquiry and contextualised ethics to analyse the humanitarian dynamics of those experiencing mental distress.

Personal Reflection and Context – I work in conflict settings that are beset by chronic and complex humanitarian crises. Some of these contexts have been embroiled in conflict for decades and the bearing witness and experiencing of violence has carried forth into new generations. As a researcher in global health, transcultural psychiatry and medical ethics, I develop trauma therapeutic interventions for conflict-related gender-based violence against the backdrop of limited mental health infrastructure and severely stigmatising notions of mental distress. Suffering, however, is fluent in the cultural narratives of poetry, literature, songs and even proverbs, which reflect the plights both of tradition and modernity. A culture's traditional ways of expression distress are fruitful for developing understanding of cultural conceptualisations and meanings of suffering. For example, this has been the basis of a traditional storytelling intervention of my current work. This has been developed alongside colleagues from various countries, with a focus on the importance of storytelling for mental health support for gender-based violence and conflict-related traumas[1,6]. Translating suffering into mental distress within health-based frameworks is a challenge, and a challenge that is not necessarily a justified battle. In other words, from an ethical point of view, I need to critically consider the ways that stories are told and received.

To this end, I share the ethical plight of the global mental health volunteer. What is the space and place of responding to suffering and distress? What are my normative values and biases, and what are my motivations? Alleviating suffering may appear as a benevolent response, yet good intentions are not necessarily sufficient for an ethical justification of intervention. I recall a conversation with a colleague several years back. She asked – and I must say, out of generosity and concern – what she could do to help my colleague in one of these conflict-affected cities. I was struck by her conviction that there was something she could do to relieve the psychological burden of my colleague, a woman enduring systematic and structural gender discrimination and violence as well as threats and risk to her life on the basis of her work in women's mental health. Could she, in fact, be able to provide any such help? Perhaps we could say 'no'.

What then could a global volunteer in mental health do to alleviate the suffering that is borne from enduring the crisis and which is generating the need for psychiatrists and other mental health care professionals?

Identifying the 'Ethical' Roots of Medical Volunteerism in Mental Health

Volunteer psychiatrists and mental health professionals are typically volunteering in a particular capacity. This relates to their prior education and training. Often this has been in western psychiatry and in a high-income country. They then seek to embark on a short-term voluntary position in the context of a limited mental health infrastructure. Due to such limitations of mental health care, placements may be attached to non-governmental organisations (NGOs), or to clinics rather than psychiatric hospitals or outpatient/community mental health care. Whilst medical volunteering has been critically viewed as motivated from harmful notions of victimisation (in that local people serve as a means to meet volunteer's needs, or for the right reasons but ignorance and ill-preparedness harm the intended beneficiaries, often without volunteers' grasp of the damage caused), there is also potential to fulfil ethical principles that underly the right reasons, namely, 'the spirit of solidarity, social justice, equality, and collegial collaboration'[3].

General medical education curriculum in the Global North typically contains at least some elements of global health. The notion of universalism in medical practice has been sustained through growth of innovation and knowledge of diagnosis and treatments. In parallel, there is greater recognition of health from a rights-based approach, which generates theoretical justifications for moral approaches to improving the right to health, or the right for an individual to flourish. Such is the capability approach (to be healthy) put forward philosophers such as Sridhar Venkatapuram[8] who writes:

Of the four broad categories of factors that affect, determine, influence, produce, cause, or constrain ('cause') a person's functioning and longevity, there is something especially and uniquely troubling when social arrangements cause human beings to suffer preventable impairments or to die prematurely. In contrast to an individual who suffers a physical or mental impairment resulting from playing a dangerous sport that she freely chose to pursue, or even the case of a person born with an unpreventable nor treatable genetic disease that leads to a shortened life burdened with severe impairment, there is something particularly alarming when the onset and experience of impairments and premature death are linked to social arrangements in the production, persistence through generations, levels, distribution patterns or differential experience of impairments and death is a moral worry of a different kind. It is a worry that individuals have been wronged in some way. It is a worry that relates to justice.

The ethical impetus, then, for responding to suffering in global settings is in part recognising the wider structural forms of injustice as well as the needs of the individuals experiencing the crisis.

Global Mental Health Movement as a Humanitarian (Ethical) Endeavour

The Movement for Global Mental Health (MGMH) has served to address the treatment gap and burden of disease due to mental illness. The treatment gaps between those who require mental health treatment and those who do not receive treatment are significant throughout vast swathes of the world. There are two fundamental principles of the GMHM, which also ground the ethical principles that are derived from the ways that GMHM can be effective. These principles are namely 'evidence on effective treatments and the human rights of people with mental disorders'[7]. The GMHM inherently is an antidote for the ethical violations that occur to individuals with mental disorders, including abuses of both physical and psychological well-being, denial of rights to receive care and freedom[7]. There is a global landscape, then, of a mental health crisis, and the response of psychiatry is a humanitarian response regardless of whether the country is suffering from a disaster or conflict. It can therefore be said that all acts of volunteering in psychiatry are humanitarian events, and that there will be certain situations that are burdened with multiple and intersecting crises. The result is that the ethical weight of the volunteer is further highlighted given that there is a magnified risk of harm as well as potential benefit for the recipients. The high need for mental health care during and in the aftermath of disasters and conflict also provides 'a unique opportunity to scale up care to the affected population' (ibid.).

However, the standardisation of a global *mental* health has received various rebukes about its very notion. The idea that the mind can be understood through a universal paradigm is highly contested. To what extent then can a volunteer trained in a dominant biomedical paradigm of psychiatry be able to capture the cultural nuances of mental health that are shaped by existing socio-political-historical narratives, and will play a role in the vulnerability of an individual when considering the long-term clinical management of mental health care? Similarly, the implementation of diagnosis and assessment against the backdrop of limited available therapies is also likely to limit the role of the volunteer. It is important to consider the ways that a volunteer's mental health training programme critically analyses the particular skills and lenses that are needed to equip volunteers with the ethical reflexivity to identify the complexity in meanings of diagnosis.

Transcultural Trauma and Normative Values in Suffering

Although psychiatry is a broad discipline, trauma is inherent in the situations that lead to mental illness. The narratives in communication and conceptualisation are the locus of the psychiatric formulation. The space for these narratives needs to be gained and earned and cannot be a result of a simple clinical interview.

To overcome this potential fracture between benefits and harms in the moral landscape of volunteering in psychiatry, the importance of our values becomes ever more pertinent and poignant. This has been advanced by Fulford[5] in his initiatives to create a values-based practice in psychiatry. To translate Fulford's vision into an international and global perspective, it could be that the new generation of volunteering in psychiatry will be a union of value-based belief systems. The ethical impetus of the volunteer psychiatrist is to navigate their own value-laden world to self-perceive their cultural viewpoints that are often projected into the *Other* in the transcultural ethical encounter. To this end, we may need to reframe the paradigm of suffering and what it means to respond to that suffering in the work that we do to receive and respond to stories of suffering[2]. The limitations of psychiatry become highlighted during times of crisis and conflict, and to fulfil the principle of 'do no harm' may redefine the identity of the volunteer psychiatrist, which Peter Hughes elegantly points out in his reflections of volunteering during humanitarian crises in Chapter 18 (whereby he partakes in planning funerals rather than prescribing).

Conclusion

Volunteering in psychiatry is a channel for keeping the moral conscience alive and many of the issues that volunteers are confronted with are replicas of the philosophical dimensions that continue to besiege psychiatry in any capacity or locality. It is a form of recognising suffering. However, despite the attempts to receive and respond to suffering borne from crises and conflicts, including the humanitarian crisis of global mental health treatment gaps, a renewed reflexivity is required amid the ethical shadows of practising psychiatry as a volunteer. The harm of an uncontextualised ethics needs to be prevented. Recognition of the ethical encounter is as crucial to managing mental disorders as much as medication and other therapeutic forms of psychological intervention. Volunteers working in mental health require adequate skills and training in cultural, ethical, reflexive and values-based practice, otherwise the MGMH will be overshadowed by the need for a globalised medical ethical movement. A good intention does not necessarily translate to a good outcome, unless the good intention is to be ethical.

References

1. Ahmad A. Taking on the Taliban: Ethical issues at the frontline of academia. *Bioethics.* 2019; *33*(8), pp.908–13.

2. Ahmad A. and Smith J. (eds.). *Humanitarian Action and Ethics.* London: Zed Publishers; 2018.

3. Bauer I. More harm than good? The questionable ethics of medical volunteering and international student placements. *Tropical Diseases, Travel Medicine and Vaccines.* 2017; *3*(1), pp.1–12.

4. Bloch S and Pargiter R. 2002. A history of psychiatric ethics. *The Psychiatric Clinics of North America.* 2002; *25*(3), pp.509–24.

5. Fulford KW. Values-based practice: a new partner to evidence-based practice and a first for psychiatry? *Mens Sana Monographs.* 2008; *6*(1), p.10.

6. Mannell J, Ahmad L and Ahmad A. Narrative storytelling as mental health support for women experiencing gender-based violence in Afghanistan. *Social Science & Medicine.* 2018; *214*, pp.91–8.

7. Patel V, Collins PY, Copeland J et al. The movement for global mental health. *The British Journal of Psychiatry.* 2011; *198*(2), pp.88–90.

8. Venkatapuram S. *Health Justice: An Argument from the Capabilities Approach.* John Wiley & Sons; 2013.

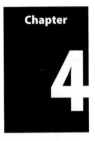

Ethical Issues in Global Volunteering: Practical Considerations

Sophie Thomson, Peter Hughes and Sam Gnanapragasam

Overview

The overarching principle of ethical volunteering is to 'do no harm'. Volunteers need to think carefully about how to behave, and what to teach and how to discuss ideas. There have been examples in the media of volunteers in charitable positions behaving inappropriately, including sexual exploitation of vulnerable people, and these cause huge suffering, trauma and humiliation to individuals and organisations. Nowadays organisations have strict safeguarding rules. It is critical to stay professional at all times.

Volunteers can find themselves in difficult situations, often beyond clinical training and experiences encountered in the UK. Sometimes, there can be impossible choices to make. There are grey areas in different societies that need further discussion with local hosts to be better informed on how best to proceed. Discussion with experienced colleagues and responsible agencies on an individualised basis is a wise and necessary approach.

Further, there can be significant ethical issues with volunteering in countries where there are violations of human rights (e.g. female genital mutilation, gender-based violence and child abuse). Sadly, abuses are common in some countries, and these can raise ethical dilemmas. Questions arise, such as these:

- Should you participate or stay away?
- What can be done to help?
- Should you speak out?
- Would raising concerns make more trouble and cause more harm to the people with mental illness?
- What should you do if you find serious violations once you have arrived in a placement? Although it can be right and appropriate to say what is not acceptable, sensitivity and diplomacy will help sustain a useful discussion.

Common Ethical Themes

There are a number of key ethical themes that are important to proactively consider prior to, and during, global voluntary placements. This is not an exhaustive list, and indeed consideration here does not mean that you will face all of these challenges. There are no easy answers to these issues and advice and discussion are usually needed with local partners and colleagues to understand key cultural context and nuance.

Human rights – Clinicians and trainers face situations where abuse of human rights needs attention. There are countless ethical issues here, for example the rights of women to make their own decisions about their health; physical and psychological abuse of mentally ill people; lack of confidentiality; and access to health services for those with disabilities. It is always important to have a human rights-based approach and speak out.

While we can offer advice on some of these things, it is best to talk through with colleagues how they can solve their own problems and to do this in an appropriately sensitive way. Offering a human rights perspective on practices can be very helpful to health care practitioners. However, no one likes to be lectured and told they are doing something wrong. Solutions must come from our hosts and working with patients and their families. Volunteers need to understand that it can be very difficult when people work in a very challenging environment to have even the basics of a private room for a clinical consultation.

Poverty – The disparity between the volunteer's situation and the grinding poverty of so many people in the world is stark. There are sadly no easy fixes. It is considered a necessary minimum to be reflective and mindful of realistic professional objectives. The circumstances may also feed into broader motivations to take action. However, there is a need to be careful to exercise self-care – to some degree, it does not help to take other people's problems home and protecting oneself aids the ability to be appropriately useful.

Politically challenging countries and regimes – Working in politically sensitive countries where human rights may not be respected is a fraught area with no clear answers. Different organisations will have differing views. Some organisations may err on the side of neutrality to ensure access under the humanitarian flag, whilst others may be more proactive in speaking out and/or advocating for certain positions. There is always a balance to be sought and advice needs to be taken on this.

Gender – Gender is a profoundly important issue in global working. Gender-based violence (GBV) is alarmingly high. There are forced marriages and FGM (female genital mutilation) in some contexts. Women may have less access to health care. Mental health care may be degrading and stigmatising.

Neo-imperialism – It is important to consider the historical and contemporary context of global volunteering. For a UK global volunteer, there is the ethical issue of possible neo-imperialism, being the 'white saviour', and 'imposing western principles' on the rest of the world. It can be a difficult power dynamic that needs reflection and continuing attention throughout a piece of work. It is necessary to work in partnership and on an equal footing, and with the use of global principles and materials. Volunteers need not be embarrassed or ashamed of the great opportunity for training they have had and can share. Well-trained professionals from around the world have a lot to give but they must have the right attitude and seek to learn, and each must recognise the limits of their own knowledge and competence. For example, encouraging south-to-south volunteering where volunteers may come from regional/neighbouring countries rather than high-income countries can provide a rich source of learning.

Pharmaceutical industry – There are clear ethical standards in the UK for dealing with the pharmaceutical industry. Accepting gifts or samples is not accepted or encouraged. Training in the UK brings familiarity with scrutinising details of clinical trials, clinical studies and attention to possible side effects of medications. These same principles need to be followed globally, especially when educational opportunities are limited, and health workers' professional development is often reliant on pharmacological industry paid events. There can also be issues of affordability of medicines that are promoted as opposed to older/generic medicines that people can afford.

Brain drain – This is a huge ethical challenge. Trying to lessen the drift of skilled health workers to high-income countries needs attention. Some ways have been to focus on training other cadres such as medical assistants, clinical officers and midwives. These health workers are not doctors. They have usually done a specific course on health, generally over three or four years. Some of these professionals can specialise in mental health. For different reasons, they are less likely to leave their countries and may be more likely to stay in their home areas than drift to the big cities. Messaging needs to be clear, ethical and sustainable: If health workers wish to travel, it should be to gain experience to take back to their country of origin. At the same, it is necessary to recognise that these people are human beings with complex relationships and individual liberties and have the right to make their own decisions. Hopefully, through your support in volunteering and training, colleagues who are trained will feel motivated to stay and give back to their country or return after further studies, but it is not the place of visiting volunteers to be judgmental about their decisions.

'Voluntourism' – Volunteering tourism is described as people travelling to areas for their own curiosity and interest and, in doing so, creating a market that the local economy/system needs to cater for. For example, in volunteering in orphanages, in some extreme cases, this has been linked to young people and children being forcibly placed (even kidnapped) into orphanages to meet this demand. There are key ethical issues of sustainability to consider in this area, although it is also important to recognise that, for some, the initial voluntary experience may be a gateway into more conventional and sustainable ways of volunteering/capacity building.

Time-limited placement – Volunteering is by definition time-limited. This creates a fundamental conflict. The question is: what happens afterwards or when the funding ends? Has the work made any difference? Will it last? Ideally, volunteering should be for long periods, even years, to make a sustainable change. In this book, projects are described that worked to make sustainable changes in relatively short periods of time through various strategies, including the incorporation of virtual learning and partnership development.

Common Ethical Scenarios

This section outlines a number of commonly encountered ethical scenarios and sets out the considerations needed when facing these.

Scenario: Human Rights Abuse

Example: An older person is tied to a tree as part of their management by her family, to control her difficult and challenging behaviour. You meet the patient in this situation, as part of your mental health work, and you have a discussion with the family. They speak of their desperation to care for their mother in a remote conflict area. Prior to this, the patient would repeatedly run away towards places of danger. The family tied her up with compassion and care, although, as an outsider, it appears awful to you.

Discussion: An immediate instinct is to untie the patient. However, in this example, it became clear that this would lead to further harm and even death if the patient ran to the front line of the conflict again. The patient was not immediately untied, but the family committed to regular health worker reviews. The patient was given a depot medication for untreated psychosis and, after some time, the family were able to untie the patient. The patient no longer ran away as the paranoia was now treated.

Scenario: Governmental Violation and Speaking Out

Example: You note discrimination or even abuse by the government organisations and forces towards particular communities. This may include verbal, physical or sexual violence.

Discussion: One of the challenges of working in countries with known governmental violations of human rights is finding a way to separate the work from the government or organisations abusing their power. A common example is discrimination against the LGBTQ+ community. This often will come up naturally in a training event. Many charities and international organisations manage to make it clear that providing assistance neither condones nor supports the actions of the government in the country where they are working. Unfortunately, there is always a risk that a country may close its doors to you if you are seen as too critical, and a balance needs to be found. As volunteers, we have a duty to speak the truth, but we also need to recognise that it is not within our remit 'to change the world' during the placement. We all need to carefully reflect on what is appropriate, and we should seek advice within our organisations and volunteer governance structures.

Scenario: Racial or Political Discrimination

Example: You are asked to treat one group of patients and not the other on account of the political situation in the country. This may overlap with religion, ethnicity or other socio-demographic characteristics. Or you may be asked to treat a loved one of a political leader rather than other patients due to social position.

Discussion: Where possible, you should be consistent with the principle of treating all individuals fairly and equitably, based on need. Examples where this may not be possible include a threat of violence to yourself or others. At times, there may be local customs and ways of working to understand and adhere to, and this should be considered with your supervisor and local colleagues.

Scenario: Gender

Example: You have diagnosed a woman with severe depression and want to prescribe a short course of antidepressants. Her husband is suspicious of western medication and says he does not agree with this. She would like treatment but cannot go against her husband's decision.

Discussion: In some places, women do not have the right to make decisions about their own health and wellbeing. For example, in some countries the husband may have to consent even to a Caesarean section as she cannot. The rate of possible obstetric complications, including fistulas, can be high. Fistulas are an example of a condition with many mental health and stigmatising societal effects. This plays out with mental health care as well. Women are at increased risk of mental health problems but face obstacles to accept mental health care. Local clinicians are more likely to know what might work to help women receive appropriate treatment, who may be best able to persuade related male decision makers, although sometimes this may not be possible. Volunteers need to be very aware of gender issues and ensure that this is a strand of all work.

Scenario: Brain Drain

Example: You are asked by local colleagues with whom you deliver teaching about how best to, and for your help to, emigrate and work in the United Kingdom healthcare system.

Discussion: It is important to be considerate and empathetic to the needs of your local colleagues and people you teach/train when they ask for your help. Whilst you have an obligation not to further outward migration, this does not mean you should react in a hostile way to the desire to emigrate. It may be worth having a discussion regarding the motivation for this, as at times this may be related to push factors (e.g. lack of pay, lack of career progression/training opportunities or risk to self/family in the current system) or pull factors (e.g. pay and work conditions). This will help you determine how best to support the individual, as well as the wider system. It might be framed as gaining particular experiences in the UK, such as the Royal College of Psychiatrists' MTI scheme, before returning to give back to their home.

Scenario: Applying/Imposing UK Model of Care

Example: You come across a treatment-resistant patient who you feel would benefit from Clozapine medication. However, the local care providers do not feel it is the right prescription.

Discussion: Whilst it would be possible to prescribe Clozapine, and indeed there may be a strong clinical rationale, it is important to consider the implications that this might have on the individual, the wider system and the sustainability when undertaking/advising such an act. For example, the medication itself is expensive (most health systems are out of pocket, so this has implications for the individual and family), and the requirement for the monitoring of blood tests and so forth would also have an added expense. Further, there may not be a system for monitoring in place and, as such, they may not get the required monitoring both in terms of blood tests and in terms of medication review by health professionals. Therefore, it is important to be careful when seeking to apply UK models of health prescription or treatment and to consider the local context and sustainability of such practice.

Scenario: Pharmaceutical Industry

Example: During a training session you come back from a drug company-sponsored lunch and find that your training flip chart has been replaced by an advertisement about vitamins that treat anxiety.

Discussion: Teaching sessions, including those sponsored by pharmaceutical companies, often provide the only professional development opportunities locally. Participants enjoy coming to meet friends and learn about important clinical developments. At the same time however, companies can easily skew accurate information to sell their products. Taking time to review safe, informed prescribing may help. Following international guidelines such as mhGAP can help overcome inappropriate prescribing.

Scenario: Inappropriate Behaviour in Colleagues (e.g. Sexual Misconduct by a Fellow Volunteer)

Example: You note that your colleague has been using sexual workers locally, and you are unsure how best to respond.

Discussion: It is important to note that this is not ethical and most non-governmental organisations and charities have a strict code of conduct relating to such activities. There is usually mandatory training before starting any work. This should guide you in what to do and who to speak to. It is a very important issue in global work. It is necessary to follow the guidelines of whichever organisation you are with or get advice from your supervisor.

Scenario: Poverty – Should You Help?

Example: You see a patient or a family struggling to get the care needed due to a lack of money. You wonder to yourself whether you should pay for the treatment yourself?

Discussion: This is no doubt a challenging situation and scenario. In some ways, there is no right answer, and while there is a natural inclination to support the individual in front of you, it is important to take a step back and recognise the sustainability of reacting to each situation and the role of charity in your placement. At times, giving money may also foster an unhealthy dynamic with you and the patients you treat, as well as wider colleagues. Indeed, the system needs justice not charity and, as such, the wider work you are doing in trying to build a better system in a sustainable manner is likely to yield results in the longer run. An exception to this might be through the principles of Psychological First Aid (please see Chapter 9). Here, there is a focus on dealing with basic needs.

Scenario: Rest, Guilt and Impact on Clinical Care

Example: There are a number of patients requiring clinical care and support. You are due a rest day and are unsure whether it is right to be off duty, as doing so may result in patients not receiving the care they need, and so may even face death or prolonged suffering.

Discussion: This is no doubt a challenging and difficult scenario. On the one hand, you have been doing a lot of work across many days and so have made a considerable contribution, but on the other hand, a period of rest will mean some may not receive care during that period.

Firstly, it is not possible for any person to work 24 hours, 7 days a week. Indeed, it is not advisable and would be unsafe.

There is a need to ensure that your own well-being and safety is maintained. In the longer run, despite the difficulties faced, you need to be able to look after yourself where possible so as not to add burden to the system locally, and so that you can sustainably contribute to the field of global volunteering going forward. If you are tired, stretched and have not had adequate rest, it will be harder to make decisions, it will impact your judgment and you will indeed make mistakes. It may sound stark to say that people may even face death when the volunteers finish for the day, but this is a real example. The volunteers may struggle to finish their day's work without feeling angst-ridden. However, it is not fair or ethical for your peers or patients in those contexts to work beyond normal human endurance. This applies to both the UK and overseas and is especially important in emergency situations. This scenario underlines how it is helpful and necessary to consider having a supervisor (possibly one based locally and another based in the UK) to help you during the placement. The identification of supervisors or mentors should ideally happen before the placement.

Scenario: 'Separate Lives'

Example: You find yourself living in a privileged context with good accommodation, security and a 'safe' compound where local care workers/colleagues are not allowed to visit you. At the same time, you note that many of your colleagues, and the development sector more broadly, all go to nice restaurants (expensive and out of reach to the local community) and appear to be living a parallel life to the local population.

Discussion: There is not an easy answer to this. For employees, international staff are paid much more than local people and lead a much nicer life than those national staff with whom they work. It is not really possible to immediately change the rules that impose these separations. What can be done is to work hard, respect all colleagues and beneficiaries, respect human rights, relish the treats that are allowed and, at the same time, acknowledge personal challenges made by leaving families and home comforts in choosing to undertake the placement. Volunteers do need to tolerate complex emotions and conflicts.

Scenario: Time-Limited Volunteering and Leaving

Example: As you near the end of your volunteering trip, you feel that although you have made progress, the overall situation has not changed hugely and there are still large parts of your project to be completed. At the same time, you are due to return to the UK due to existing training needs, job demands or other family/caring circumstances.

Discussion: This situation is difficult and, indeed, it can be normal to feel guilty at this stage. This underlines the importance throughout the placement, starting from the pre-placement stage of planning, to think through the sustainability of the project and how to ensure that broader project aims are met going forward, without you. It is important to monitor and evaluate a project (see Chapter 11), as even if it does not meet the aims, there is much learning that can come out of the process for the local community and yourself.

Conclusion

Global volunteering can be an immensely valuable and rewarding experience for all stakeholders, if undertaken in an ethical manner. Volunteers may find some ethical dilemmas more troubling than others and it is not uncommon to be deeply moved by particular patients and their situation. It can be frustrating at times, and therefore there is a need for companionship and supervision. Whilst many volunteers may find the resources and support to cope, others may need special help to work through their experiences.

Benefits of Global Volunteering to the United Kingdom

Peter Hughes

Introduction

The UK has benefited hugely from health workers around the world coming to work in the National Health Service (NHS) and care services. This started in the colonial era and has been continuing since then due to a mixture of push and pull factors. Looking at hospitals, GP surgeries and care homes, it is noticeable that staff come from all over the world. In fact, what is one of the biggest ethical dilemmas is the 'brain drain' of doctors and nurses from where they are needed in low- and middle-income countries (LMICs) to the UK and other high income countries[3]. Given this unequitable movement of the health workforce, there is a moral obligation on the UK health system to support LMICs. Global volunteering helps somewhat in redressing the balance, although it should be seen as one small component and not a replacement for systemic workforce shortages.

With strained health services in the UK, particularly as highlighted during the Covid-19 pandemic, there is a need to justify global work and prove that working globally benefits the UK and improves the workforce in the NHS and/or social care sector. This reflects a significant change in the volunteering philosophy over the past few decades. Increasingly, the emphasis is on partnerships that benefit both the UK and partner countries[5].

This chapter considers the benefits and challenges of global volunteering on the UK health system. This includes a review of notable literature, programmatic evidence and personal reflections.

Global Volunteering Benefits to the UK

Global volunteering is of benefit to the UK in not only meeting the moral obligation, but also in enhancing the skills of the individual care provider and organisation after a project is completed. There are a number of notable publications that articulate the benefits of global volunteering.

History and Notable Literature

The Global Health Partnerships Report written by Lord Crisp in 2007 – '"The UK contribution to health in developing countries' – highlighted the benefits of global volunteering to the UK and raised this practice on the agenda[6]. This report has been very influential and has led to much reflection and to professionalisation of volunteering.

It discusses global learning and how to incorporate this back into the NHS. It illustrates that global volunteering is an opportunity to enhance education, skills and knowledge throughout the world and back home in the UK. Volunteers can develop skills in countless ways including those related to leadership, confidence and clinical practice. In addition, global volunteering can improve the reputation of the NHS and the UK and meet the moral obligation of mutual benefit. Lord Crisp also mentions the soft diplomacy of global volunteering in improving bilateral national relations. There have also been governmental discussions of how volunteering may lead to economic benefit to the UK through development of trade and closer relations.

This report and new approach led to the Global Exchanges Programme supported by Health Education England. This organisation supports global volunteering for staff from the NHS with an implicit expectation of benefit back in the UK.

'Turning the world upside down' was a concept that was furthered to embrace the co-development model and challenge outdated colonial notions of one-way knowledge transfer[7]. It articulated the benefits of learning from innovations in LMICs and applying them in the UK to improve patient care. This is crucial with increasing budgetary pressures on NHS practice and the need to adapt continuously to this.

There have been many examples of where the UK and the NHS can learn from global innovations. For example, simple technological mobile phone-based practices in India that give health messages are easily translatable to the UK. There is also the example of an educational programme for schoolgirls in Jamaica to improve their well-being. The world is now globalised and there can be an easy transfer both ways of innovation in health and social care.

WHO mhGAP[8] is an example of an approach that was designed for training in LMICs but can easily be translated to UK practice. mhGAP has been mentioned much in this book for international work and there is no reason why this could not be used in UK as well. mhGAP is a WHO initiative to enable increased mental health access in LMICs through task shifting and strengthened integrated primary and mental health care[9]. Many UK volunteers have been advocating for mhGAP principles to be used in UK primary and secondary care. The Volunteering and International Special Interest Group of the Royal College of Psychiatrists (VIPSIG) has been running weekend orientations since 2011 for a UK audience. This is for people to familiarise themselves with skills for global mental health but implicitly there is also an expectation of them using these skills in their own NHS practice.

Since Lord Crisp's report, there has been a Report by the Academy of Medical Colleges on Volunteering[10] and the All-Party Parliamentary Group on Global Health on 'Improving Health at Home and Abroad Report'[11]. These highlight the benefits of global volunteering in UK and worldwide.

Skills and Development Domains

UK global volunteers are thought to benefit from having improved skills in reviewing pathways of care, service integration, commissioning, leadership and teamwork. This is affirmed by Lord Darzi's Next Stage Review[12] which highlights hard skills related to education, leadership and languages and also clinical skills that accrued from global volunteering. Soft skills that were identified included flexibility, resourcefulness, confidence and patience. The other area of learning is using technology that is cheap and adaptable in the NHS.

Global volunteering can be very helpful in terms of recruitment and retention in NHS trusts when they have programmes of global partnerships[13]. At a time of great strain on mental health services, this is an important pull factor to make jobs more attractive and help to retain motivated staff. Whilst there are issues of backfill, the advantage of a refreshed health worker back from volunteering is that clinicians may be more motivated to continue in their NHS job. Often after volunteering, people are reflective of the advantages as well as the challenges of the NHS.

NHS Trusts have identified the benefits of global volunteering to the UK. The NHS Confederation states that 'NHS staff volunteering overseas experience these frugal innovations, but support and processes often aren't in place to facilitate sharing them with colleagues and the wider NHS'[14].

The Framework for NHS Involvement in International Development 2010[15] published by the UK government sets out several key benefits to the UK of global volunteering:

- Personal development
- Professional development
- Helps recruitment and retention
- International profile, connections and networking

In addition, there were also benefits related to:

- Enhanced training opportunity, at low cost to the organisation
- Staff morale
- Enhanced reputation of the organisation, which promotes recruitment and retention
- Corporate social responsibility that can lead to enhanced performance and sense of job satisfaction
- Culturally appropriate NHS services
- Improved patient experience, for example in terms of transcultural skills of the health worker

There have been formal evaluations of the benefits of volunteering upon return to the UK. A Voluntary Services Overseas'(VSO) survey of returned management professionals showed that 80% believed that they gained expertise that would not have happened in the UK[4]. Similarly, the Royal College of Psychiatrists (RCPsych) have undertaken evaluations and found similar findings (see case study below). See Figure 5.1 for how skills gained in volunteering have been applied on return to the UK. See the Case Study for narrative reflection of the voluntary experience.

Challenges for Volunteers Returning to the UK

There have been some challenges reported of volunteering globally and its effects upon return to the UK[16]. These included financial costs with accrued debt on return to the UK. There can be a loss of earnings and pension during a period of absence and beyond. Sometimes people have had to work with locum agencies until established back in their career. Volunteers may also feel clinically deskilled on return to their former NHS job, and they may need some support during the reintegration process.

Another challenge is related to lack of formal and professional recognition in the UK of global voluntary work. VIPSIG at the Royal College of Psychiatrists advocates for volunteering to be recognised as a professional asset when health workers are seeking

Ask patients

- 'What do you think has caused this problem?'
- 'What makes you or the problem worse or better?'
- To learn and use breathing exercises every single clinical day
- 'Who or what is there to support you?'
- 'How do you spend your day?'
- Check understanding and expectations

Interventions

- Every clinical encounter has some explanation component
- Cover mental, physical, social and even spiritual health
- Understand culture and ask colleagues and family to explain what might be different to your own
- Patient is in charge of treatment/at the centre and should be directing their care
- Human rights are a fundamental principle in every encounter
- Always involve families and value their input
- Always be gender sensitive
- Always check on the welfare of children of patients and elders

Management

- It is always about people first in any leadership context
- Listen to people
- Plan any interventions systematically
- Involve all stakeholders in any decisions
- Always write down everything and do formal reports
- Be the first to realise if you are wrong and listen to criticism

Figure 5.1 Learning from global work that has been applied in UK practice

employment back in the UK. The Ghana trainee programme of the RCPsych was approved for training, which demonstrated that working globally has an intrinsic value for training in the NHS (see case study below).

Case study: Royal College of Psychiatrists (RCPsych) Volunteering Scheme

The Royal College of Psychiatrists, as further described in this book, has had a volunteering scheme since 2005[1]. This has led to around 100 volunteers working on assignments since its foundation. A particular focus of the volunteering scheme is on psychiatry trainees and enhancing their professional development[2].

One of the programmes has been the Ghana trainee exchange. This is described further in Chapter 21. In this programme, trainees in higher psychiatry travel to Ghana for three months to work in a comparable job to their own in the UK. These three months have been recognised for training back in UK. Getting this approval was a feat in persuading the General Medical Council, Royal College of Psychiatrists and the Educational Deanery that the overseas experience would benefit the trainee in their UK training. The program has debriefed all the doctors who went to Ghana and surveyed their perception of benefits to themselves and their work in the UK.

In 2015, the volunteers' scheme of the Royal College of Psychiatrists was surveyed to look at the benefits to the UK of volunteering as well as other aspects of the experience[16]. The results match other surveys of health workers such as by VSO[4].

The RCPsych survey on benefits to the UK of global volunteering found that volunteers felt that their work overseas had helped the NHS. There was a high perception of being able to use skills of teamwork, leadership and transcultural skills. Next were clinical skills, resources, time management, management and innovation. Less strong were academic skills, and audit was lower in terms of skills acquisition and transferable to NHS. There was a deep dive into some specific cases of volunteers. They reported how useful the experience was for consultant interviews, and professional, personal and academic life. One person used the experiences to start a mentorship programme. Another was able to use psychodrama back in the NHS.

There was one negative account of a volunteer's experience which related to environmental issues of housing and heat, but this person still valued the professional development and was able to use this back in the UK.

There are some volunteers who have a negative experience, and these clearly will not bring a benefit to the UK. These are few. For some it may relate to a change of physical environment (e.g. heat, insect infestations or accommodation). It may also relate to becoming homesick, and missing friends, family and other support structures. There may also be project-related challenges and mismatch of expectations. Fortunately, this is increasingly rare with more open selection, training and supervision of volunteers. For every voluntary assignment, there needs to be a plan for when things may not be working out. Even those who have not had a positive experience will often still say that they could understand the benefit of global volunteering, even if it was not right for them.

Case Study: Personal experience and reflections

Herein, I write as one such volunteer and reflect upon the impact my global work has had on my UK work.

I am a psychiatrist in the UK and can say that my global work has moulded my practice and has been transformative personally and professionally for me. It has been immensely satisfying to be able to bring what I have learned in the NHS to overseas work and to apply what I have learned globally to the UK. The downside has been the tension between working in a job I love in the UK and working globally.

I identify strongly with all the survey results of volunteering described above. I have learned to be a leader, make decisions collaboratively and chair important meetings. I have also learned how to work quickly and adapt to fast-changing circumstances in emergencies.

There are some negative aspects back in the UK that I have faced, including financial loss, pension loss and missing out on professional opportunities due to physically being away. It can take a while to adjust back to life in the UK after an assignment. It can be frustrating not to have all my skills learned overseas utilised in the UK. During one six-month placement abroad, I came back to find that my NHS job had changed, and I had to return to a different role.

Clinically, I feel that I have learned at least half of my professional skills from my global work. There, I learned the vast majority of my psychosocial skills. I have been able to share these skills through teaching others. There are countless examples I can think of where my global work has helped me become more culturally competent and understand my patients better wherever they have come from.

Every day, in my clinical work in the UK I use the VIPSIG Psychological Toolkit as described in Chapter 9 For example, the hand technique is something that I have found immensely useful. This leads me to ask my patients better questions.

UK Volunteering

Those who volunteer globally often also volunteer locally (either before or after the global volunteering work). Examples include:

- **The Helen Bamber Foundation** has been supporting refugees and others in the UK in different iterations since 1985. It began as 'Freedom from Torture'. This is supported by UK volunteers working with survivors of extreme human cruelty such as human trafficking, domestic violence and ill-treatment because of gender or sexual orientation as well as with survivors of torture.
- **Medical Justice** has volunteers supporting refugees. It was started by a refugee and supports those in detention in the UK.
- **Doctors of the World UK** supports free GP services for refugees and asylum seekers. This includes much mental health care.

Volunteers have spoken of how their work dealing with refugees and asylum seekers is their most satisfying role professionally. When they speak of someone getting residency and not having the fear of deportation, they describe a great sense of satisfaction and joy. Up and down the country there are so many other examples of volunteering. Mental health professionals give educational talks or volunteer with Rethink, Samaritans, refugee drop-ins and many other examples. Retirees work hard providing all types of useful volunteering work.

Key messages
- Global volunteering benefits the UK NHS
- There are hard and soft areas of benefit
- It is a factor in enhancing recruitment and retention in the NHS
- There is much volunteering happening in UK at grass roots level

Conclusion

Almost every volunteer will say how the experience has enriched them personally and professionally. To help understand how to translate benefits to NHS organisations upon return, it is helpful for the volunteer to be versed in the related literature and consider the experiences of those who have undertaken similar placements. There is a need to further research benefits to the UK[17] so as to continue demonstrating the benefits to the NHS of global volunteering. This will help ensure that people working in the NHS are more readily released from their work and supported to go away, as well as return refreshed and skilled up. Advocacy that ensures global work is professionally recognised needs to continue. Also, efforts to enhance recognition of the rewards that volunteers bring back from volunteering need to include removing professional barriers on return. The NHS needs to learn as well how to make most use of this valuable resource.

References

1. Royal College of Psychiatrists. Global volunteering scheme of the Royal College of Psychiatrists.

2. Hall J, Brown C, Pettigrew L et al. Fit for the future? The place of global health in the UK's postgraduate medical training: a review. JRSM Short Reports. 2013;4(3):1–8.

3. Gureje O, Hollins S, Botbol M et al. Report of the WPA task force on brain drain. World Psychiatry. 2009;8(2):115.

4. Machin J. The Impact of Returned International Volunteers on the UK: A Scoping Review. London: Institute for Volunteering Research; 2008.

5. Syed SB, Dadwal V, Rutter P et al. Developed-developing country partnerships: benefits to developed countries? Globalization and Health. 2012;8(1):1–10.

6. Crisp LN. Global health partnerships: the UK contribution to health in developing countries. Public Policy and Administration. 2008;23(2):207–13.

7. Crisp N. Turning the World Upside Down: The Search for Global Health in the 21st Century. CRC Press; 2010.

8. World Health Organization. mhGAP intervention guide for mental, neurological and substance use disorders in non-specialized health settings: mental health Gap Action Programme (mhGAP). World Health Organization; 2016.

9. Hughes P, Thomson S. mhGAP – the global scenario. Progress in Neurology and Psychiatry. 2019;23(4):4–6.

10. Academy of Medical Royal Colleges. Academy statement on volunteering. AoMRC London; 2013.

11. All-Party Parliamentary Group on Global Health. Improving health at home and abroad: how overseas volunteering from the NHS benefits the UK and the world; 2013.

12. Darzi A. Quality and the NHS next stage review. Lancet (London, England). 2008;371(9624):1563–4.

13. Cox J. UK International Health Links Funding Scheme (IHLFS). International Psychiatry. 2010;7(4).

14. NHS Confederation. Leveraging the experiences of NHS staff volunteering overseas; 2020.

15. NHS and Department of Health. Framework for NHS Involvement in International Development 2010. https://severndeanery.nhs.uk/assets/Internationalisation/TheFrameworkforNHSInvolvementinInternationalDevelopmenttcm79-26838.pdf.

16. Tyler N, Ackers HL, Ahmed A et al. A questionnaire study of the negative outcomes for UK health professional volunteers in low and middle income countries. BMJ Open. 2020;10(6): e037647.

17. Tyler N, Chatwin J, Byrne G et al. The benefits of international volunteering in a low-resource setting: development of a core outcome set. Human Resources for Health. 2018;16(1):1–30.

Chapter 6

Preparation for Global Volunteering: Professional, Personal, Psychological and Practical

Sophie Thomson

Introduction

Preparation is the key to an impactful, satisfying and sustainable experience for both volunteers and hosts. This chapter outlines important considerations when preparing for a global volunteering placement by attending to the four Ps of preparation: professional, psychological, personal and practical. See Table 6.1.

1 Professional Preparation

Finding a Suitable Project

The voluntary journey starts with the decision to volunteer your skills and your time. It may be that the ethos and work of a particular charity appeals, or you feel that you want to work with a smaller organisation that specialises in a particular area of interest. Or maybe you

Table 6.1 Preparation for global volunteering

PROFESSIONAL	Decide what you want to do and select a placement
	Check safety and security advice and protocols
	Agree roles and responsibilities with volunteering organisation or plan and agree objectives with hosts
	Prepare materials and training needed for the project
	Prepare appropriate evaluations
	Finalise preparations with hosts
	Arrange supervision and attend pre-trip briefing
PERSONAL	Work with family and friends on arrangements for time away
	Arrange time away from work or training
	Learn about destination, culture, language, national priorities
PSYCHOLOGICAL	Reflect on personal expectations and aims
	Reflect on personal coping strategies
PRACTICAL	Organise health check and vaccinations, visa, money and insurance (see checklist in Appendix 2)

want to go somewhere you have never been before and explore working in an entirely new setting. Perhaps your own skills, background and cultural knowledge lead you to want to work with colleagues in a particular area and you feel inspired to try to set up a project. Acknowledging to yourself what really motivates you will guide you to exploring appropriate possible volunteering opportunities, keep you focused on what matters and help sustain you during the tough times. You may wish to refer to Chapters 3 and 4 which discuss some of the ethical considerations and motivations in global volunteering.

Having decided what you want, you may well find only limited possibilities from advertised vacancies in large organisations that accept volunteers within your available time frame, so you may need to decide if you are prepared to try something new. Many non-governmental organisations (NGOs) and charities prefer longer-term commitments than working health professionals can manage and some prefer applicants to have had previous exposure to international work. Smaller charities and NGOs may offer more flexibility. Other schemes such as The Royal College of Psychiatrists' volunteering scheme have developed short-term training experiences to help College members participate in international volunteer work. Although these are each relatively short commitments in time, they are usually in the context of a longer-term project. You will find examples of this volunteer work in later chapters.

To aid your search for international volunteer opportunities, please see the opportunity list provided in Appendix 1. Listed organisations include Global Health Exchange (Health Education England)[1], Mental Health Innovation Network (MHIN)[2], Mental Health and Psychosocial Support (MHPSS)[3], Médecins Sans Frontières (MSF)[4] and Tropical Health and Education Trust (THET)[5]. These organisations offer resources and information. They provide up-to-date reports of international projects and helpful guidance, as well as some possible volunteering opportunities. Faith-based organisations such as PRIME[6] also offer volunteering opportunities with the chance of sharing a common outlook, training experiences and organised team support. There are other organisations offering volunteering opportunities online. However, these may have variable suitability for mental health professionals and discernment is required. It is worthwhile checking carefully that what is expected from volunteers matches your skill set, interests and time available, as well as the ethical and practical arrangements of organisations or individuals asking for volunteers.

It is inadvisable to work in isolation. Working, and particularly travelling, with a team provides personal and professional support, a chance to learn more and have company. An established charity usually means a warm welcome, a clear pathway to productive relationships and programmes as well as protocols to follow.

If at all possible, find out as much as you can by speaking to someone who has been to your chosen country and has been part of a project previously. Do your research by finding reports from any previous volunteers as well as sourcing up-to-date information that is available online, including travel and anthropology articles and books and ethnographic research.

Finding global opportunities can be an uphill struggle. Many doors can close before one finally opens. It can take a lot of 'door knocking'. Unfortunately, a definitive list of up-to-date opportunities is not possible as the world of global mental health is dynamic. The Covid pandemic has limited many opportunities. At the same time, it has expanded digital global volunteering possibilities and increased the number of potential exciting online options.

It may be helpful to join a network of volunteers such as the Volunteering and International Psychiatry Special Interest Group (VIPSIG)[7] of the Royal College of Psychiatrists, or the equivalent in your professional body. These organisations can help you develop your own personal network with like-minded global volunteers and be part of developing new opportunities. A growing list of resources can often be found through such networks.

Ideally, volunteers from psychiatry should hold a Membership of the Royal College of Psychiatrists (MRCPsych), or have other equivalent professional qualifications, and have several years of clinical work experience before volunteering. However, core trainees in psychiatry, or more junior mental health professionals, can also be volunteers and there may be opportunities suitable for them. One example is the King's Somaliland Partnership[8], where a junior trainee was paired with a more senior psychiatrist to deliver training to medical students in Somaliland.

Whatever you decide to do, it is necessary to ensure that it is a secure and safe situation and that you only sign up with an organisation with robust planning, professional standards and appropriate support. The Foreign, Commonwealth & Development Office (FCDO)[9] has reliable and regularly updated information about many aspects of travel to all countries around the world. Political and geographical changes can unexpectedly occur and keeping an eye on the FCDO website helps understand the possible risks of travelling to, and within, countries and how to access help if needed.

Developing New Projects

Building a new project begins with making links with interested national or international colleagues. Finding an international colleague with an interest in partnering can be difficult. At present many projects begin with chance meetings at training events or national and international congresses such as the Royal College of Psychiatrists International Congress. Clinicians born or trained outside of the UK may have advantages by knowing key people working in mental health in their country of origin. Knowing the culture and language as well as how mental health systems work can also be a great advantage – see the following case study

---

Case study of Royal College of Psychiatrists' projects

Two of the most successful recent volunteering projects under the Royal College of Psychiatry volunteering scheme were built by motivated College members. They were international medical graduates with a knowledge and understanding of both the UK and their original homes in Kashmir and Myanmar. After contacting old friends and colleagues, they organised the practicalities and invited other College members to join small training teams to travel with them to provide training packages in mental health. These are described in Chapters 12, 13 and 20. Many other College members have also been making contact independently with international colleagues and providing training, mentoring and support that is much appreciated, especially during the Covid pandemic.

A good working relationship with partners is vital. International colleagues may not know what we can offer, and we may not know what they would like to offer us. Sharing knowledge, experiences and expectations with partners can lead to a realistic plan with shared objectives. Ultimately, a volunteer needs an invitation to a host country. Volunteers will be guests and need to remember this.

It is possible to do an excellent small project without formal funding. Small charities and some local fundraising can help and sometimes produce surprising generosity, as well as helping to spread the word about the benefits of your proposed project. Applying for a grant for a project is usually done through an organisation, but a small team can apply. It means doing some homework to find out what is available at any given time. An example is Tropical Health & Education Trust (THET)[6], which offers small and large grants on a regular basis, usually for specific countries.

Setting up a new project may take considerable time, but seeing a project through from an initial vision to a satisfying improvement in services for people with mental illness can give a sense of purpose that may not often be experienced whilst working within the NHS. However, the reality is that some new projects do not come to fruition and a volunteer may find themselves doing something quite different, having learnt a lot along the way. Nevertheless, there is an increasing appetite for international training supported by the Royal College of Psychiatrists' new 2020–2023 International Strategy[10] and closer liaison with international colleagues in the near future is likely. This will hopefully produce more opportunities to create bespoke projects.

Planning with Hosts

If you volunteer with a large medical-based NGO, you will be given a mission manual, with checklists, protocols and guidelines with pre- and post-mission support, all based on years of experience. For all organisations, especially smaller NGOs, you will be wise to check that you understand and are comfortable with all the arrangements.

If you are organising a volunteer project for yourself or a small team and have formed a working partnership with a host organisation, you will now need to find out as much as possible about their expectations, resources and culture. This will bring you to a more realistic place to discuss what you can and cannot do, as well as continuing to build a mutually respectful working relationship. Previous volunteer experiences suggest that sometimes expectations can be quite unrealistic, both for volunteer and host. Continued communication helps to ground a realistic plan. You may be asked to do something different on arrival. You will need your diplomacy and negotiation skills to work towards agreed objectives, so sorting these out ahead of time is advisable and sharing written agreements helps.

Co-production means that there can be less of a power dynamic and more mutual learning. You cannot expect to be an expert on a local health service and culture even if you are from the diaspora. As best you can, you need to make yourself aware of local services, national policies and possibly other issues such as drug supply and national stakeholders, so that a decision can be made about what might be needed for a sustainable outcome.

Exploring what is already known and what potential participants or organisations want to work on begins to craft a useful mutually agreed programme of work. It may be possible to have a blended project bringing together online and face-to-face work. This is becoming a good model for sustainability. Blended work allows for the initial co-design of the project online and then good partnership experiences during a visit, as well as continuing to share learning and support and possibly supervision after a trip. Increasingly, sharing of appropriate articles, books, videos, online courses and pre-prepared materials electronically enables people to work at their own speed and enjoy more interactive, workshop-style meetings, when and if face-to-face meetings are possible.

Even with a well-organised plan, you will need to be ready to adapt your expectations. As a simple example, some volunteers may expect participants in training events to follow UK ideas of timekeeping, dress codes, ways of speaking and learning, and respect for the value of evidence-based research. In one volunteer trip, the participants arrived throughout the morning and chatted a lot. This was normal behaviour for them and they meant no disrespect. In another country, participants were seated quietly and attentively in their chairs at 8 a.m. and did not want to ask questions. Breaks for meals and prayers at times are vitally important in some countries and an interest in evidence-based services is new to some people.

As well as training, volunteers may be asked to do tasks such as writing up proposals, auditing, research, quality improvement projects, health record-keeping, programme organisation, clinical supervision and many others. You may even find yourself on local media and giving interviews. Many volunteers have learnt new skills in all of the above areas. Be prepared to do something new and skill yourself up.

Types of Volunteering Placements Available

The common types of volunteering placements are listed in Box 2.

Types of volunteering placements available

Different types of voluntary placements that arise include:
1 Humanitarian mission
2 Teaching, training and capacity building
3 Clinical service delivery
4 Service development
5 Research

Humanitarian Volunteer Missions

Sometimes opportunities come up in humanitarian settings. Particular care may be needed in deciding if these opportunities are appropriate, as living conditions may be really difficult and the work required not entirely clear. A greater range of skills may be needed, and you could find yourself doing any number of tasks including situational analysis and response, administration, teaching, clinical work, supporting staff or joining others in whatever needs doing. Self-care is very important in humanitarian settings. Going with a large organisation with firmly established procedures and protocols aligned with local services and government plans is essential in humanitarian work. Lone volunteers, no matter how well meaning, can easily get in the way and they can actually have a frustrating and unproductive experience. This is one area where working alone is entirely inappropriate. This is a particularly challenging type of work. It involves being part of a team and following clear internationally agreed guidelines. Chapter 2 on humanitarian work has further guidance and there is a continuous professional development e-learning module on this issue on the Royal College of Psychiatrists' educational site.

Teaching, Training and Capacity Building

Often the most helpful and commonly requested task a UK volunteer can undertake is the delivery of training. This may be with delivery of a pre-arranged training programme such as the WHO mhGAP or a more bespoke programme based on local needs. Please see Chapter 8 for further information about the preparation required when delivering a training programme.

Clinical Service Delivery

Agreeing to do clinical work needs to be carefully planned and works best with longer-term projects. It is usually not advised for short-term visits as volunteers may not have enough time to learn the way local services work, nor understand the cultural norms and clinical presentations, and consequently face the issue of looking and behaving like an outsider. However, engaging in clinical work may be appropriate when there is a crisis and an absence of human resources. This is a substitution of services, not a support. The ideal, however, is to support clinicians in increasing skills and capacity. Ideally seeing every clinical encounter as a training opportunity may help local skills development.

In longer-term projects, the traditional model of learning medicine by apprenticeship and supervision may work well and give much more opportunity for ongoing learning for both volunteers and host clinicians. Volunteers can help train clinicians in skills and knowledge that will last with 'on the job' training. It can be laborious and time-consuming when the trainer sits in with the health worker in their clinical work, but it is effective if it can be done for a sufficiently long time. Sitting in on a clinic in primary care or a psychiatric clinic can be hugely illuminating by helping to explore diagnostic options and psychological treatments. For example, in primary care clinics worldwide there are many patients with psychosomatic conditions, missed depression and anxiety syndromes who could benefit from simple psychological interventions.

Registering with the national equivalent of the General Medical Council and arranging medical indemnity will be needed for making clinical decisions and taking clinical responsibility. You will be beholden to the rules and regulations of that country when practising and hence checking you are comfortable with these is advisable.

Service Development

Scoping and working with colleagues to understand what already works and what might work better in the future takes skill and time and is best suited to larger projects with governmental and other stakeholder support. Experience in the UK and other higher-income countries may not necessarily be helpful and there may be a lot to learn from how people in resource-poor areas manage.

However, the volunteer can make huge contributions even without specific training. Examples include the development of community and home treatment services and models of early intervention adapted to local circumstances. There is much to learn from stakeholders' reflections on lessons learnt from the UK development of governance structures, policies, documentation, diagnostic coding and a myriad of other areas both clinical and non-clinical.

Service development involves developing local professional relationships and working with local committees. But there may also be times when you need to present to the minister of health or their representative. You may be required to sort out budgets and write bids for money for new services. It is crucial not to replicate UK services but to co-design models adapted to local needs and what is appropriate for that service. It is very important to have participatory consultation about service development, incorporating service user and civil society representation. Examples of service development are setting up new clinics, super-vision systems, new hospitals and developing training structures. In Sierra Leone (see Chapter 16) the volunteers there were involved in all of these service developments and in applying for new funding.

Academic Development: Research and Curriculum Development

Support and encouragement for academic development can help clinicians and managers understand that every country has an important contribution to make to the international bank of knowledge and skills. The open access publication approach can ease financial barriers, but busy clinicians may have trouble finding time to do research, and finding funding can be a challenge.

Volunteers can use their experience to foster interest and skills for academic work, audit and research as well as curriculum development and the preparation of clinical protocols and guidelines. Publications on global mental health and the contributions from low- and lower-middle-income countries (LMICs) could soon change the face of international mental health work for all. Such projects should be undertaken in partnership and co-development, and, indeed, joint ownership and authorship is the best way forward.

Preparing Materials and Evaluations

Preparing lectures and gathering resources such as PowerPoint slides, videos, journals, questionnaires and interactive learning techniques may take considerable time as it will often mean adapting work that has originally been prepared for UK purposes. It may be important to search for new global mental health information and advice about appropriate cultural adaptation. Engaging hosts and participants in discussions about a work plan and programme with these resources will help make an appropriate and useful project.

You may need to enquire about interpreters if your own first language will not be understood in the host country. Contact with your interpreters ahead of meetings with your host may help decide how best to work together.

Preparing how the work will be evaluated, measured and reported needs to be agreed with stakeholders, especially if the project is funded by donors. Donors will expect a clear monitoring and evaluation strategy and report. Even if the evaluation is very formal or more informal, it is always necessary.

At the very least, the professionalised volunteer should always be evaluating their work and producing a report at the end as this is an important tool for ongoing work and sustainability. See Chapter 11 for further discussion about monitoring and evaluation.

Establishing Supervision and Support

However senior and accomplished you might be, you will value support. Regular contact with a mentor or supervisor enables responsible practice and helps when facing problems which are complicated by many factors outside established clinical and teaching experience and culture. Ideally you will not be alone, and you can be supported by working in a team or even a pair, which is so much better than struggling on your own. But if you are working alone, and do not have the chance to speak regularly with a UK-based supervisor, there are usually other possibilities, such as meeting with other local expatriates and new colleagues in your placement. Psychiatry trainees based in the UK will need to establish their supervision as appropriate with local postgraduate deaneries and schools. It may also be possible to work with an approved supervisor who is a co-trainer overseas. There may be supervisors available through other professional colleges and in the United Nations or international NGOs.

Finalising Preparations

Agreeing the Programme with Hosts

The day will come when getting a complete plan written and agreed with partners moves the project into the final preparatory phase. A document summarising agreed objectives, a day-to-day timetable, evaluation tools and practical arrangements helps everyone to know how the programme will (hopefully) work. As an example, after much discussion and sharing with hosts, the Myanmar project team of six UK-based trainers worked for two days to finalise a 15-page document to be sent to host colleagues for final comment and appropriate amendment. Large projects will clearly require considerable consultation with involved stakeholders and supporters.

Preparing for a Global Mental Health Project: Connecting to Hosts online

When working with hosts electronically preparations may need to be different as volunteers will not usually have the opportunity to meet with international colleagues in a personal way before and after meetings. It can be easy to miss cultural cues and planned interactive work may be hindered by the capacity of the internet connectivity. However, it does mean that more detailed planning is possible with the option for quicker, more frequent online meetings at very little cost.

Pre-trip Briefing

A good briefing with supporters in the UK prior to travel is essential, as checking as much as possible sets the stage for realistic expectations and achievable goals. This should include how to prepare the '4Ps' of Preparation: Professional, Psychological, Personal and Practical (see Table 6.1). As well as a thorough professional briefing, common personal concerns at pre-trip briefings include problems about managing in unfamiliar situations, internet availability, homesickness, loneliness and adequate preparedness.

2 Personal Preparation

Personal preparation includes preparing yourself and your family and friends as well as making arrangements for work responsibilities and how you will most comfortably re-enter life back in the UK when you return.

Organising time off through study leave or unpaid leave, as well as time out of a training programme, are possibilities. Some professionals opt for a 'gap year' out of usual work commitments and others may be fortunate enough to have a sabbatical.

Important as it is, volunteers can easily get distracted by professional needs, like going off to an academic conference. International volunteers can lose track of the need to plan to live and work in a very different environment where resourcefulness, flexibility, cultural awareness and communication are important skills for success. Even experienced travellers can find adjusting to a new culture challenging. This time you are not a tourist but a guest, and you have to establish and maintain a working relationship with new colleagues, as well as living in a new environment. Adjusting to living in a culture with social norms different to home, possibly different religions, a potentially troublesome political environment, a different historical background, different food, different ways to spend spare time and different beliefs, takes time, adaptability and genuine curiosity. Spending time learning about the people, culture, national priorities and the history of the place you will be visiting will make it much more interesting for you, as well as showing your hosts your genuine interest and respect for their lives and work.

Phases of adjustment have been described as 'honeymoon', often followed by a phase of negativity and, finally, adjustment. 'Culture shock' can be ameliorated by working with known colleagues, preferably a team who have prepared together, and having an awareness of stereotyping, communication skills and a sincere interest in how other people live their lives, especially how they manage in their different resource settings.

Volunteers can have surprises in their responses to working away from the familiarity of home, friends and familiar comforts. For some, going to a new culture can be a profound and transforming experience. For others, it is a refreshing and engaging time away from usual responsibilities. Some people simply don't enjoy it. Yet even if that is so, they usually don't regret that they tried it. Doing humanitarian work probably makes more demands on peoples' resources and hence the need for working with an experienced organisation.

Women volunteers may need to accept that they might be treated differently in settings outside the UK. Reflecting on how to deal with this may influence the choice of where to volunteer and inform decisions about how to manage it. Once again, a good understanding of cultural norms and what to expect helps, and a decision to live within different cultural practices may actually produce an important learning experience.

3 Psychological Preparation

Reflecting on how to prepare psychologically and spiritually might include considering how you usually manage stress, what your strengths and supports are, what annoys and frustrates you, how you cope with risks, and what gives you satisfaction and pleasure.

Some people find it helpful to write down lists of their expectations. Reviewing your motivations and aims as you move along the preparatory journey may help you clarify realistic expectations and keep your focus on achievable goals for yourself, your family and the people you will be joining in the international work.

Hopefully your family members will be supportive, and you can continue to be in contact with them electronically, and you can get home quickly if really necessary. Consider what they might need whilst you are away.

4 Practical Preparation

If you take a position with an established organisation such as MSF, MHIN, UN or even the smaller NGOs, you will probably be given what you need or at least a checklist of essentials. Even so, it is wise to check on what might go wrong and double check you are as ready as you can be. It is necessary to be ready for what can go wrong (see Figure 6.1).

1. No one being at the airport to meet you on arrival
2. Accommodation not being ready or appropriate or you can't find it
3. Losing money or property. You can be seen as a rich foreigner and an easy target for theft
4. Your hosts asking you to do something completely different to what you had agreed. You need to use negotiating skills and be flexible!
5. Your hosts not keeping to objectives or changing the programme unexpectedly
6. Participants not engaging with training or supervision or not being interested in working on sustainability
7. Not having a training venue sorted appropriately
8. No one turning up for your training
9. Saying the wrong thing (e.g. insensitive or political)
10. Other volunteers trying to 'save the world'
11. Becoming substitutes for local services
12. Losing boundaries in friendships
13. Falling out with friends or team
15. Getting exhausted or burnt out
16. Getting ill or having an accident
17. Loneliness, boredom and homesickness
18. Abuses of alcohol, drugs and sex
19. Re-entry back into the UK not being well-planned
20. Not asking for help when you need it

Figure 6.1 Practical things that can go wrong for a global volunteer

Health Considerations

There are a number of health-related considerations pre-departure. These include:

1 Health Advice, Vaccination and Malaria Prophylaxis

See a travel consultant. Get vaccinations and medication well ahead of time. The usual suggestions are to make sure you have the standard UK vaccinations, then decide what you will need for the specific area you will be visiting. The travel consultant can tell you exactly what is needed.

There are several good travel websites that can help. An example is Fit For Travel (fitfortravel.nhs.uk/home)[11] which is NHS-based and often used by international volunteers. It gives details about diseases to consider and preventive measures to be aware of. It can be hard to decide just how many vaccinations you might need, and it will depend on your current state of health, where and when you are going and how much risk you are prepared to take. For example, rabies vaccinations may be important if you are going to rural areas a long way from good rabies immunoglobulin supplies.

Yellow Fever vaccination is mandatory in many countries, and you will need to prove you have had this with your yellow vaccination record card. If not, you may need to pay an expensive fine and get a vaccine at the airport or even be turned back in some countries. The Yellow Card or the Carte Jaune is the international certificate of vaccination and prophylaxis and is the equivalent of a medical passport.

Malaria is the one that everyone should think about. It can kill. Do not risk it. Follow the advice and do everything you can to avoid getting malaria if you are in an endemic area, especially during high-risk seasons. Take anti-malarial medicatons properly. Wear long sleeves at dawn and dusk. Use DEET anti-insect spray. Make sure that wherever you go there is a mosquito net (or take one) and get netting over the windows. Any fever during or after your visit could be malaria. There are reports of volunteers getting malaria months after a trip even after taking prophylactic medication properly.

2 Dental

Have a dental check. Toothache is one of the most horrible things to happen in the field. Going to a local dentist is best to avoid where possible. If you need to see a dentist, find out where the United Nations (UN) or NGO staff go for treatment.

3 Reading Glasses

Bring a spare set of glasses. Ideally bring your lens prescription in case you need new glasses. Ensure you have sufficient contact lenses and fluid. Sunglasses are useful in many countries.

4 Identify Good Hospitals with Emergency Services

It is worth finding out what health care is available where you are going and have their number in your phone. Find out where UN and international partners go to clarify pathways to care. The services will likely be private so make sure you have enough 'emergency cash' or a credit card to pay up front.

Ambulances vary a great deal, and you are highly unlikely to find anything remotely resembling what we have in the UK in many LMICs. You may be asked for a cash payment for transport.

5 Travel Insurance

Get reputable travel insurance, one that includes repatriation to the UK (medical evacuation). No one ever thinks they will need this until they do. Unfortunately, accidents and illnesses happen more than you might imagine. Being ill overseas can be extremely worrying.

6 Road Safety

Road traffic accidents are an increasing problem internationally. Do wear a seat belt. Consider refusing to use a dangerous vehicle. This is by far one of the biggest dangers for a global volunteer.

7 First Aid Kit

Pack a first aid kit with more than bandages, plasters and paracetamol. It is often possible to buy medication over the counter in LMICs but there is a huge business in fake drugs in some countries so you might have to pay high prices for brands you recognise, and hope that the drugs are real and in date. So, it is worth taking extra supplies of all the medication you know you will need (perhaps duplicate) and keep at least one supply in your hand luggage when travelling. Your personal medication is one of your most valuable possessions. Also consider asking your travel consultant for the latest medication for severe diarrhoea and buccal medication for vomiting. The chance of getting tummy trouble at some stage can be high, even if you are very careful. Taking a supply of antibiotics is worth considering too. Tea tree oil works as antiseptic and anti-itch and has the added bonus of smelling great.

Some people take their own needles and intravenous-giving sets, especially if going to an area with high HIV rates. Masks and sterile gloves are easy to pack. Condoms are worth taking, for friends, if not yourself.

Do not take any controlled drugs. Take a doctor's letter if these are absolutely necessary.

For humanitarian emergencies you may be given a first aid kit containing all of the above in a convenient pack.

8   Fitness – Physical and Mental

Get fit. Being in good basic physical health will help you enjoy the whole experience. Check if you are in a place of high altitude as this will need acclimatisation. If you have underlying health conditions, you may need to think carefully about where you offer to travel or even whether it is wise to go at all.

The same is true for psychological health. There will probably be stresses in the environment, the weather, sharing facilities, as well as unexpected events.

Consider what can be your support – preferably something that needs no equipment, like yoga or meditation, and also electronically-loaded reading material and family photographs.

Loneliness can be a problem. Try to learn a few words of the local language, at least be able to say 'Thanks'. Make an effort to talk to people. Go for walks and go to local cafes. Home sickness can be common, but by the time you are ready to leave you may well wish you could stay longer.

9   Risk Assessment

Do your own risk assessment. What could happen and what would you do? Try to talk with someone who works, or has worked, in the country and get the truth about risks. Make an emergency plan in case something serious happens, for example next of kin contact details, insurance information, special requests, etc.

10   Common Health Problems

The most common health problems that UK citizens encounter overseas are:

o   Gastroenterological problems such as traveller's diarrhoea. Rarely does it progress to more serious problems. Basic standards of hygiene, health and safety are often not mandatory, legal or enforced in many places. Think, and wash hands, before you put anything in your mouth. Remember the common saying: 'If you can't peel, boil or cook it, forget it!'

o   Slips, trips, accidents and falls.

o   Heat intolerance. UK volunteers are often not used to drinking the amount of fluids needed in really hot climates. Also sunburn when people do not wear suitable clothing and hats.

o   Bites, stings and wounds that easily get infected in humid climates.

o   Recurrence of pre-existing injuries and illnesses under stress.

Documentation and Paperwork

There are a number of key documents and paperwork to have in order before departure. These include:

1 Passport which is valid for at least six months. Keep a copy somewhere safe as it speeds up replacing a lost passport.
2 Visa(s), which may take a long time to obtain.
3 Registration with the local medical regulatory board/General Medical Council equivalent if you are doing any clinical work. This can take time. Remember that you will be bound by the laws of the country where you are practising.
4 Medical indemnity/insurance. 'Good Samaritan' emergency work can sometimes be covered but it is best to check with your insurer. If you are doing regular clinical work, you will need to get special indemnity cover. Check the situation, particularly in humanitarian emergencies where your host organisation can advise.
5 Letters of welcome to your work carried in your hand luggage. You will probably need these on arrival.
6 Address of first hotel/accommodation, also needed on arrival.
7 Contact details of the person meeting you on arrival.
8 Copies of your own contact details, emergency plan, your GP number and contact details for any specialists you consult. Copy everything to team/colleagues and family. Photograph it all or keep printed copies with valuables.
9 Fill phones with ICE (In Case of Emergency) numbers and other important numbers.

Packing Your Bags

Remember you will probably be carrying them, so pack as light as you can and do not take valuables/jewellery. Use tough rough-looking bags with the name and address of your destination clearly marked inside and out and photographed in case they get lost.

1 Personal

Clothes suitable for the weather and culture are needed. Lightweight, easily washed, hard-wearing clothes that cover most of the body are advised. Long sleeves and long pants for malaria protection as well as cultural respect should be strongly considered. If you are doing a professional job, you need to look professional and deserving of the respect that will be shown to you as an international guest representing your charity, Royal College or organisation. You will need at least one good outfit and comfortable walking shoes. Other items to consider include:

o Raincoat and something warm for cold nights
o Mosquito net, if appropriate
o Long-sleeved tops. Shorts for home but not for outside
o Bathroom needs – more than enough for your stay
o Toilet paper, sanitary needs, soap and towel. Hand gel for emergency handwash
o Torch and penknife
o Water bottle and water purification tablets (saves plastic)
o Spare glasses and sunglasses
o Hat with brim

o Electric plug convertors (at least two)
o Padlock for bags and moneybelt
o Gifts (e.g. key rings/pencils/books/postcards/sweets)
o 'Can't live withouts' – such as photos, entertainment and electronic books

2   Professional

o Laptop loaded with your own and team members' prepared work
o Charger and link to PowerPoint
o Power/ battery pack
o Memory sticks
o Handouts
o Copies of training material sent ahead – simple, well-written, up-to-date, interesting and in basic English (check if hosts can print them)
o Pens markers or whatever you use
o A second phone for local SIM and in case of theft, loss or poor charging access
o Hard copies of manuals and books for teaching (e.g. WHO mhGAP)
o Soft copy of Psychological First Aid and other key materials
o One or more copies of 'Where there is No Psychiatrist' which has very useful information and can be used as gifts[12]

3   Money

Credit cards and cash, preferably US dollars or euros, with enough for emergencies, carried in at least two separate places. Small denomination clean bills from within the past ten years. UK pound sterling may not be accepted.

It is usually best to avoid changing too much money at the airport but do change a small amount for the next couple of days. Work out how much will be needed for tips in local currency and have some extra notes available (e.g. US dollars in small denominations). This is important for arriving at the airport where you may be hounded by porters, whether you want one or not. It can be difficult finding a convenient ATM in remote places and even in cities it may be difficult to find a working machine. Your hosts can advise you of where to go for an ATM. If you do plan to use ATM machines, consider looking into bank accounts that allow free withdrawal overseas. Beware of illegal money changers and black market traders who may offer you fake or outdated notes.

4   A Sense of Humour, Patience and a Ready Smile!

Please note that there is a tick box version of the packing list in Appendix 2.

Conclusion

Preparation is key. The more the better. Remember the 4Ps – Professional, Personal, Psychological and Practical. Clarify your self-motivation for volunteering and use this to identify a suitable project. If seeking to develop projects, engage in co-development with local partners and diaspora groups. Personal preparation can be aided by speaking to those who have previously volunteered in a similar situation to where you will be going. Personal considerations relating to expectations when away, maintaining relationships with loved ones and reintegration are necessary.

References

1 Health Education England.Global Health Partnerships www.hee.nhs.uk/our-work/global-engagement.

2. Mental Health Innovation Network. www.mhinnovation.net.

3. Mental Health and Psychosocial Support Network Mental health and psychosocial support https://app.mhpss.net.

4. Médecins Sans Frontières https://msf.org.uk/.

5. Tropical Health Education Trust. www.thet.org.

6. Partnerships in International Medical Education www.prime-international.org/home.htm.

7. Royal College of Psychiatrists Volunteering and International Special Interest Group (VIPSIG). www.rcpsych.ac.uk/members/special-interest-groups/volunteering-and-international.

8. King's Health Partners – King's Somaliland Partnership www.kingshealthpartners.org/resources/case-studies/21-kings-somaliland-partnership.

9. Foreign Commonwealth and Development Office. www.gov.uk/government/organisations/foreign-commonwealth-development-office.

10. Royal College of Psychiatrists International strategy 2020–2023. www.rcpsych.ac.uk/docs/default-source/members/international-divisions/rcpsych-international-strategy.pdf?sfvrsn=b0dda422_6.

11. NHS Scotland. Fit for travel. https://fitfortravel.nhs.uk/home.

12. Patel V, Hanlon C. *Where There Is No Psychiatrist: A Mental Health Care Manual.* 2nd ed. Cambridge: Royal College of Psychiatrists; 2018.

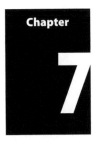

Onsite: Working in Another Country

Sophie Thomson and Peter Hughes

Introduction

This chapter explores the practicalities of arrival in another country, settling in and co-working with hosts in final planning and preparation for programme delivery. The importance of spending time getting to know the people with whom you will be working as well as the flavours of the world they live in will help shape a meaningful collaborative experience. Self-care and care for the team remain a constant theme and an important point of emphasis.

Arrival and Getting Settled

The initial period will entail recovery from the journey, meeting new colleagues and exploring the logistics of what happens where you will be working. Host welcomes vary from quick introductions and hotel drop-off to visiting local homes, medical associations, meeting important local dignitaries and visiting local places of interest. Usually, hospitality is exceptionally good. You may be nervous about meeting your hosts. Don't be. You will be treated with great respect and hospitality and be seen as a representative 'ambassador' of your home country and profession.

Airport Arrival

There will almost always be someone to welcome you at the airport, or there will be a plan for a taxi to take you to your accommodation. If there is no one to meet you, just be ready to make your own way to your accommodation. Make sure you have the full and accurate address of where you are staying and your workplace. Ideally have this written down as your electronic devices may run out of battery or, due to geo-locks, you may not be able to access all of your applications. Have several phone numbers for your hosts and WhatsApp contact details, and always have enough money for a taxi and hotel for a night. Get a local SIM card as soon as possible and call your hosts.

Accommodation and Living Conditions

Standards of accommodation vary around the world and most volunteers accept humble basic living conditions and do not ask for anything more. This can be very country specific. Expect power cuts as routine in many low- and middle-income countries (LMICs). Similarly, internet access may not be good or even available in a home setting, but mobile/cell phones are universal. Phone and WhatsApp may be your lifeline at home but there are towns and even cities that do not have internet. It is important to check that it is available and, if not, you will learn to adapt.

Mosquitoes are to be expected in many areas and you may need to consider this in the context of your accommodation and sleeping conditions. You are likely to have a fan to keep cool, or air conditioning if you are really lucky. Shops may be very limited and expensive, especially those that cater to expatriates. Bring more money than you think you may need.

Check with people who have been onsite before. Boredom on days off on extended assignments can be a real problem. In many countries one of the main forms of entertainment is alcohol but obviously it is important not to indulge in excess. In other countries, alcohol use may be taboo. Bring your own entertainment, such as games and reading material. Consider preloading your computer with teaching material, films and programmes before you go. Bandwidth may not be enough to download YouTube, videos, music, e-books. Toilets and bathing arrangements can vary from what you are used to at home and might be a water tank and hole in the ground in a discreet place. Running water may not be a given and hot water might be limited, or not at all accessible. Many countries may not provide toilet paper or soap. Attending to your own personal hygiene including showering is an important part of self-care. Keep washing your hands, especially before you eat.

Food

The food is likely to be what the local people eat and not necessarily to your liking. Vegetarianism can be considered unusual in some countries, but your hosts will usually adapt and try to support your needs. Be careful what you eat, as standards of hygiene may not be regulated in the same way as in the UK and you don't need gastroenterological problems when training! Wash your hands frequently. The staples may include bread, bananas and coffee, and these are likely to be universally accessible.

Local Society Norms

It can seem like everyone else is busily moving around efficiently, catching taxis and buses and bartering in shops, ordering food and chatting in tea shops and generally getting on with life. Enjoy it but be aware of the dangers too. Trust your instincts. Your hosts can brief you. For some volunteering trips there may be a formal security briefing. Some organisations request that an online security briefing be completed before arrival. The security advice is crucial. It may also be imprudent to speak about certain matters. It can be normal that bribery and corruption make things happen. The term 'Baksheesh' is often the word used for the giving of money for services rendered. Knowing when and how much to offer can be puzzling for a new visitor. Many NGO and UN organisations will not countenance payments of this kind. It is best to get advice on this on arrival.

Stereotyping can lead to making all sorts of wrong assumptions about people. The crucial thing is to be aware of how you stereotype others and how you might be stereotyped. There is a common stereotype that visiting volunteers are rich and privileged. This is actually true, relatively speaking. You may get asked for money. But it is nearly always better to refuse and thus avoid the risk of setting up an expectation for the future. Saying 'no' will be respected and not affect your professional relationship. Similarly, the volunteer needs to be reflective of how they might stereotype others and address this.

There may be places that are out of bounds in your neighbourhood, and you must respect that for both men and women. Women may have to accept restrictions on travelling or even walking around unescorted (by a man) in some countries. In almost all cases it is not advisable to go out at night unless you know that a place is safe. Again, your hosts and colleagues can advise you on this.

Clothing can be a sensitive issue for both genders in some countries. There may be an expectation of formal attire in a professional setting. Wearing sandals and shorts is usually not appropriate. Women may need to be particularly careful about clothing in some countries as covering up, even in hot climates, is often expected.

Respect and dignity go beyond clothes to general attitude and having a suitable humility. Active efforts must be taken against having, and giving the impression of having, a sense of superiority (cultural imperialism) as there is always mutual learning. Indeed, there is an opportunity to learn to respect how people manage to live and work, sometimes in the greatest adversity and poverty, and still keep smiling and be polite.

In training, there may be gender issues amongst both participants and facilitators. The expectation can be that male participants lead work, especially senior professionals. This needs to be addressed so all can participate equally regardless of gender or seniority. The volunteer facilitator needs to work hard to ensure that training is fully interactive and fully participatory.

Ideally training can be best facilitated by trainers of different backgrounds, gender and approaches to training. As a volunteer, co-facilitation with local health workers in any training enables a sense of local ownership and sustainability and is recommended.

You may get invited into discussions about local politics. Although you may wish to ascertain appropriateness depending on context, by and large, it is best to remain neutral with regard to expressing opinions about local or national government, even with regard to the health service. To do so might place your hosts in a difficult or even dangerous position. You do not want to appear naïve, so perhaps use distraction and move to another topic. On the other hand, reflecting on your own country of origin may be more appropriate. It is important, however, to consider speaking about human rights, particularly how it relates to mental illness. Abuses of women and children can be addressed with care and humility. Remember that no one wants to be lectured by a foreigner on what is considered wrong with their country. This is one of the areas that stretches volunteers' diplomacy skills.

There are some organisations that specifically address human rights abuses or act as a testament to what is happening in that country. It is always a good idea to seek advice on how to approach any issue that could be controversial. There are some people who argue that volunteers need to speak out against social injustice and not condone what is wrong. This needs very careful consideration and discussion with your hosts as you could end up causing harm in naively doing so.

There have been regrettably many incidents where volunteers from other countries have engaged in exploitative behaviours including sexual. Any volunteer now must be briefed on the necessity of avoiding any such behaviour, just as they would in the UK. It might seem that this is not necessary to say but it is essential, and briefings will cover this before arrival in the country.

As outsiders you can never assume to know the local culture or context, but fortunately visitors are usually forgiven for mistakes, especially if there is a willingness to adapt. Volunteers are not lecturers or teachers, but rather facilitators in enabling and strengthening local knowledge and skills. Hosts and the participants in training become cultural navigators. Keeping ears, eyes, minds and hearts open enriches the experience and shows appropriate respect.

Diaspora colleagues, who will be people originally from a country, can have struggles with how life has changed, and the impact of this. They themselves face challenges, and it is complex even for them.

Meeting with Hosts

This is the time to fine-tune your programme. Even agreed programmes will need checking and updating. Local political or social issues may influence a well put-together project plan and changes may need to be made. Volunteers need to be flexible, diplomatic, dynamic and work in a principle of co-production. Face-to-face discussions with hosts usually clarify what is actually expected and how the work together will proceed.

You can explain how you prefer to work and discuss if this will be appropriate for the intended participants. This may need explanation, further discussion and adaptation with host colleagues.

Occasionally you might be asked to make major changes to the programme. Having your prepared written plan available will help discussions about what might or might not be possible. Get advice, if necessary, from your supervisor or colleagues in the country. You do need to expect that the plan may deviate from what was expected but there can be limits; for example, being asked to focus on seeing private patients or even being asked to move to a different speciality. If it is a Royal College of Psychiatrists' programme, there will be plenty of support to resolve the best way forward.

Overall, it is important to try and stick as much as you can to your original work plan, although you may want to consider responding to unusual requests to help out, especially in humanitarian situations; for example, sorting out drinking water or checking pharmacy supplies.

Ideally this is the time to gather more contextual information by checking with local health workers about any important clinical concerns and gaps, and the local attitude to mental illness. If there is time, check on the views of local stakeholders such as religious leaders and private sector organisations.

Potential Challenges for Hosts

Volunteers need to remember that preparing a project may take hosts considerable time, effort and money. Hosts may not understand or may be too polite to explain the amount of work involved in setting up and sustaining an ongoing project. Even if a project does well, there may be risks politically, professionally or socially. Whilst the majority of volunteering is successful, there is a need to acknowledge that sometimes it may not work.

There are lessons to be learnt from common areas where things can go wrong. See 7.1 Box for more details.

Fostering Communities of Mutual Learning and Support

Whatever the type of work undertaken by volunteers from the UK, ongoing contact remains important. One of the key areas where the UK volunteer can help during and after training sessions is to support local supervision systems and help create a culture where this is the norm. For example, having a robust system of supportive supervision is essential for the

Box 7.1 Problems that hosts have reported with volunteers – where it can go wrong

Unexpected costs on both sides

Volunteer poorly prepared

No supervision

Volunteer trying to impose UK system and thinking 'they know best'

Volunteer does not understand local culture

Volunteer wants to 'change the world'

Parachute volunteer – no sustainability – in and out

Personality issues – interpersonal conflicts, volunteer struggles with environment (bugs, power cuts, no home comforts)

Bureaucracy, for example registering with professional organisation

Media and social media – embarrassing hosts

Professional and personal misconduct – at workplace and outside

Volunteer not being road safe

Volunteer illness, for example malaria

Volunteer has to leave because of personal circumstances

integration of mental health into primary care. The UK volunteer can provide technical advice on this and ensure that supervision continues face to face, in a group or online.

Although arranging supervision, mentoring and consultation from the UK is useful and needed in the short term, it can be far more valuable to support the growth of collaborative working groups within countries. Connecting people with each other and helping to provide a space for listening to opinions and ideas that fit with local cultural realities can help initiate and sustain developments, and work with local solutions to local problems. Linking professionals electronically or by phone across geographic space can encourage useful partnerships and support. Volunteers can become facilitators of relationship-building and step back increasingly from direct contact and become more like collegiate mentors. As an example, in the Solomon Islands a system was set up of weekly phone calls between nurses on different islands, helping with solving clinical problems and giving support for isolated practitioners.

Setting Up Ongoing Evaluation

It is necessary for the UK and host team to review the project on a regular basis, whether it be service development, clinical work, training or academic, with a review of comments and feedback. See Chapter 11 for further information on evaluations.

Taking Care of Volunteers

Working in a new environment with new colleagues and possibly new material can be stressful, especially if you are the only volunteer. It can be lonely, both personally and professionally. Working as part of a team means mutual support, an arena to discuss concerns and getting help. The other links to make are with the local services, NGOs and government agencies so that your work fits with the overall plans for development. There is also a lot of support in knowing you are part of an overarching project. For example, meeting with colleagues in public health and the United Nations in the Solomon Islands helped the volunteer to focus attention on local beliefs about mental illness and the difficulties in the prison, which were part of the ongoing national plan.

The need to keep working can be overwhelming. The literature is full of advice about volunteers ensuring that they get sufficient rest, food and sleep. The catchphrase that seems to help many people is: 'My first responsibility is to myself'. The idea is that being in good shape means you can do your best work but being exhausted and upset means quite the opposite. Having a UK mentor or supervisor is recommended, which will be mandatory if you are a trainee. Even senior psychiatrists working with a good team will do well to have a structure in place whilst working and living away from their usual supports. In humanitarian emergencies it is even more crucial to attend to self-care.

Conclusion

After all the preparation, it is usually a great relief and a pleasure to be meeting with hosts and participants and working through a programme together. Sharing experiences can be enlivening and fun. Listening to stories of suffering and impossible situations can be a struggle. Admiring how people often do cope with meagre resources can be humbling, and enlightening. There is a need to consider practicalities such as those around airport arrival, accommodation, travel, food, internet connection and the local societal norms. It can be helpful to continuously evaluate individual and programmatic progress and ensure adequate self-care.

Chapter

8

Implementing and Delivering Training as a Global Volunteer

Sophie Thomson and Peter Hughes

Introduction

Training is the most common and perhaps the most useful role for a global volunteer at this stage in the development of global mental health. Once initial agreements with hosts have been confirmed, it will be time to firm up details of agreed objectives, what training package or materials would be helpful, who will be involved, details of timetabling, as well as how best to deliver the training requested by the host. Special consideration of psychosocial interventions needs to be given to any training in mental health, as these therapeutic interventions are an integral part of the management of all people with mental health conditions.

The Why, What, Who, When and How of Training

Even if you have been given a pre-arranged brief to train subjects with specific material, you may need to negotiate with your hosts about what might be most suitable for the proposed participants in the time available. Arrangements will vary depending on who is joining the training – working with psychiatrists on training in modern subspecialities, training young psychiatrists and trainees, or nurses and clinical assistants in primary care, or perhaps even organising workshops for lay people such as village elders about mental health awareness – they all need different training materials and possibly methods. However, the principle of careful joint preparation remains the same for all, even if meetings for training are electronic – considering 'Why, What, When, Where and How' should give enough information to make a suitable plan for interesting and enjoyable experiences for all (see Table 8.1).

1 Why Are We Doing This?: Objectives and Alignments of Expectations

Having a few simple but precise objectives helps to keep minds focused on achievable goals and tasks. Written and agreed objectives can relieve all concerned of feeling lost amidst lots of needs, assumptions and demands. They serve as a reference point to realistic expectations. Objectives can serve as a mission statement.

They can be as simple as engaging interest and understanding of mental health and illness, or exploring stigma in communities, learning about safe prescribing, attending to human rights or women's well-being. Discussions about objectives between volunteers, hosts and participants can be fruitful in aligning realistic expectations.

Table 8.1 The Why, What, Who, When and How

1	Why: Why are we doing this? What are the agreed objectives based on realistic expectations for the setting and time available?
2	What: What areas of training in mental health will be suitable for the participants and what materials could be used?
3	Who: Who will attending and what do they already know? Who else should be involved in organising and supporting the training to enhance sustainability? What language can be used?
4	When: What time is available? How long can the training take out of the working day and what constraints will there be?
5	Where: Where will we be working? Is there a suitable venue with adequate internet and possible air conditioning?
6	How: How can the training be most impactful and acceptable to the attendees? What methods of training will suit this project?

2 What to Train?

Hosts may have preferences for training materials. Available international sources may need adaptation for the culture and knowledge of the trainees. Lectures and PowerPoint presentations may be supplemented by video recordings, and training materials can be downloaded from the internet.

Training Materials

Training Materials to consider include WHO Training packages: mhGAP IG[1] and mhGAP HIG[2]. The WHO intervention guide (mhGAP IG) for mental, neurological and substance use (MNS) disorders in non-specialist health settings, there are few other internationally-agreed evidence-based training packages. See Table 8.2 for some of the other currently available training resources.

The WHO mhGAP IG has become very popular as it guides practitioners through an algorithmic system of diagnosis and management of common mental health conditions. It is ideal for helping experienced mental health professionals in teaching students and primary care colleagues. The WHO mhGAP IG is a 173-page printed colour-coded manual, a mobile phone app and a free download via the internet. The original 2010 version of mhGAP has now been superseded by the 2016 version 2. There are some very useful complementary short training videos on YouTube and other online video portals. This is part of the WHO mhGAP programme which was designed to build capacity of mental health care in LMICs. The advice in this book is consistent with this manual.

The WHO mhGAP IG manual is laid out with an excellent section on essential care and practice, followed by chapters on depression, psychosis, epilepsy, child and adolescent disorders, dementia, substance disorders, suicide and, finally, other significant mental health complaints (also known as unexplained medical conditions).

The humanitarian version, mhGAP HIG, is more narrative[2]. This is designed for humanitarian emergencies where there is a need for brevity and focus on stress-related conditions.

Ideally, local psychiatrists join a training team, and this helps them practise teaching the manuals and encourages good communication for later referrals of patients.

Table 8.2 Training resources

- The WHO Psychological First Aid (PFA)[3] is a useful tool to support people who are in immediate distress. It can be used by lay people and non-specialists.
- There are other WHO tools for low intensity brief psychological interventions such as Self Help Plus[4], Problem Management Plus[5], Thinking Healthy (perinatal mental health)[6], Group Interpersonal Therapy for Depression[7], Doing What Matters in Time of Stress[8] and Building Back Better[9].
- International Psychiatric Speciality Societies often have packages for training.
- World Psychiatric Association (WPA)[10] has a resource section for education.
- Scotland Malawi Mental Health Project (SMMHEP)[11] has developed a useful guide for mental health trainings, and other NGOs usually provide specific manuals.
- The MHPSS[12] and MHIN[13] websites can have valuable resources for global volunteering.
- The WHO QualityRights toolkit can be helpful in terms of assessing and improving quality and human rights in mental health facilities[14].
- There are books suitable for different levels of experience (see resource section at end of this book). The book entitled 'Where There is No Psychiatrist' takes a symptom-led approach in plain language and is welcomed by many clinicians as it can help as a training resource for non-specialists and community workers[15]. Its companion 'Where There is No Child Psychiatrist' is also very popular[16].
- There are also good downloadable materials where the training is entirely pictorial or in video form.
- There are most certainly many other publications, in book form and online, that are worthy of consideration for inclusion in training material to share.

Training the trainers in using these manuals is the current mainstay of working with psychiatry colleagues internationally, although it can also be used directly for training in primary care settings by volunteers both in the UK and internationally.

The real challenge for training with this manual is how to teach it well. It is laid out as an algorithm, which may initially feel daunting. Most UK-based mental health practitioners will be familiar with the content of mhGAP but it takes time to become sufficiently comfortable to train with the manual. Hence, the emphasis on teaching techniques is becoming an important part of UK global volunteering preparation. Participants working their way through the manual during training are helped by taking a logical approach by closely following the document, so they can practise using it. Writing notes on the manual itself helps some people.

Using the method suggested above and matching the programme with plenty of simple psychological skills training works well. Table 8.3 gives an example of a very brief programme for primary care workers based on WHO mhGAP with an emphasis on including psychological skills – this can be amended to fit the time frame available.

Undoubtedly, more evidence-based training material will become available. Digital modules and courses are currently being developed. Ideally these will be done by international working parties sensitive to cultural differences and based on research across the nations.

Table 8.3 Example of a primary care mhGAP training agenda

	Topic	Knowledge/skill
Module 1	Introduction Essential care and practice Depression assessment	Communication skills Psycho-education
Module 2	Depression management Suicide Stress and anxiety	Psychosocial support Discussing suicide Relaxation techniques
Module 3	Drug and alcohol misuse Organic conditions and epilepsy	Motivational interviewing Management of epilepsy
Module 4	Child and adolescent mental health Dementia	Parenting tips and star charts Problem-solving
Module 5	Psychosis Unexplained medical presentations	Safe prescribing

Flexibility with Training Materials

Even with a well-prepared and agreed project plan, it is best to be ready to modify the details and timetable on the 'less is more' principle. Spending time on important local conditions may be more important than covering a whole pre-prepared plan. You may need to think about ways to adjust the timetable by deciding what to prioritise and possibly reduce your usual pace by up to a half. If you know your material well, you can trim down to an acceptable pace and suitable content.

Sometimes you may need to stick firmly to a training material. For example, if working on WHO mhGAP you must keep to the manual. The WHO appreciates that training in mhGAP may need some cultural adjustments but substantially changing the content is unhelpful and possibly confusing for participants. Usually there are some minor adjustments needed.

At other times, trainers have to adapt and do what feels useful. You may have the opportunity to explore areas that may be important to the people in the room but are not on the 'official agenda'. You will certainly need to work with what fits culturally and the shape of local services and thereby hopefully co-create, with hosts and participants, a useful outcome for the improved well-being of the people with mental illness.

Case Study

In the Solomon Islands, the trainers were asked to teach Cognitive Behaviour Therapy to nurses in a long-stay facility. When it became clear that this was not working, the trainers switched to working with the nurses' interest in singing, dancing and storytelling groups as culturally-appropriate therapy for their residents. They also helped them with safe prescribing and record-keeping which was appreciated.

You will need to learn or revise your training material, so you know it well. As well as preparing an agreed package of training, it is usually worthwhile preparing a range of other possible modules so you feel confident that you can respond flexibly to the people you actually meet in training sessions. For example, knowing a programme for domestic violence or protection can be handy, and thinking through how to work with people about record-keeping and reporting adverse events can be useful. Psychological first aid (PFA)[3] is also a popular module, especially for frontline workers. Some participants may know very little basic psychiatry and refreshing your basic knowledge may be worthwhile. Finding out how to train in leadership, capacity building and developing networks of support may lead to some great research and learning for yourself!

Sometimes it can be very difficult to understand what may be required, especially if interested hosts do not quite know what they do not know and may simply ask to be taught 'psychiatry'. In such a situation, further conversations and a menu of possibilities might be worth discussing. It can be helpful to have an idea of the conditions that are common in that country. You can look at the WHO Mental Health Atlas[17] and AIMS reports (Assessment Instrument for Mental Health Systems)[18] to aid such efforts. These help to gather an understanding of known data about health and health systems. Asking your hosts about what mental health conditions they experience and are concerned about adds to this assessment.

Working with qualified psychiatrists and others interested in specialty training requires some thought with partners about what might be useful within their system. For example, would training in individual, group or family therapy be most appropriate if invited to teach introductory psychotherapy? Perhaps in practice, group therapy on wards may be a more useful start to psychotherapy experience for people who only work on wards with limited time available. What aspect of forensic psychiatry might be most needed in a setting where prisons have little or no access to mental health professionals? In a society where young people in a traditional society are becoming more educated and possibly more assertive, what aspect of child and adolescent psychiatry, as we know it, might be relevant? Packages of material for special areas such as domestic violence, child protection, cognitive behaviour therapy and specialist subjects like Avatar training will need to be sourced and prepared.

Some people are natural teachers, but other gifted clinicians and academics need help to develop confidence in presenting their work effectively. Helping colleagues to learn how to use interactive training methods, adapted for cultural and local needs, is an increasingly interesting area for development. Workshops are available through the Royal College of Psychiatrists and other professional organisations.

Mental Health and Psychosocial Skills Training

In delivering any training, there needs to be a balance of covering medication, physical and psychosocial treatments. Doctors may be very comfortable with delivering training on medication but less so on psychosocial interventions. The converse may be true in delivering training to nurses, social workers or psychologists. Both areas generally need to be covered and the exact balance negotiated.

In the next chapter (Psychological Techniques Toolkit – Chapter 9), there are details of some useful psychosocial interventions. For the authors, these interventions have been an invaluable asset throughout the world in training a variety of health professionals.

At the present time, one of the most needed areas of training globally is in basic interviewing skills and psychosocial support. In the UK, the current medical curriculum places great importance on providing a suitable environment, involving the person as much as possible, being respectful, friendly and non-judgmental, using clear, concise non-jargonistic words and attending to patient confidentiality. Here, one can even fail exams if insufficient attention is given to this critical area of training.

Unfortunately, these skills are often not taught in many countries. This may appear paradoxical as there is usually a lot of kindness and goodwill. However, there is often insufficient training, practice and modelling to build confidence to make these important skills part of everyday practice in the assessment and treatment in all areas of medicine. This is particularly so in mental health. It can be rewarding helping people to realise that psychosocial support is part of treatment and how much patients with mental illness value explanations, dialogue, respect, being heard and gentleness with sensitive issues. Principles and practices related to the human rights of consent, confidentiality and privacy help further facilitate this. Seeing psychosocial skills as part of the therapeutic process can take time. In one training, the team were called 'the human placebo' after focusing on this key therapeutic area.

Teaching about diagnostic criteria or definitions of disorders is relatively simple, but learning the art of good communication, showing genuine interest in the person, and having respect for all ages, abilities, genders and sexual orientations can be somewhat more challenging. It is often enhanced by workshops with an experience in role play.

There are many ways to improve psychological skills, and you may do well to gather your own list from all that is available online or draw on your own experience and find out what works where you are visiting. Experience shows that psychosocial skills can be taught and practised even during a short five-day training session[8]. Feedback from such training demonstrates that clinicians have increased confidence to start using these simple tools that do no harm and often provide something helpful other than, or as well as, prescribing medication. Medication can be expensive for families and produce worrying side effects (especially if these are not explained well), and potentially disempower patients.

Medication and Safe Prescribing

In many countries, particularly in humanitarian settings, the availability of medication may be limited, or suitable medication may not be available. Sometimes drugs are limited by cost to off-patent older drugs, and variable supply chains may dictate what can be used. Sometimes there are 'gifts in kind'. These are donated medications which are given with goodwill. However, they may be expired or be irrelevant to local circumstances. In one example of a psychiatric hospital in Africa, there were no medications for psychosis but a whole room filled a 'gift in kind' of Lamotrigine.

To add to these problems, advice from experienced clinicians and supervision may not be easily available. Information about side effects and appropriate dosages may not be available from drug companies advocating their newest medication.

Training modules on safe prescribing can include appropriate dosing of medication for various age groups and during pregnancy, common and uncommon side effects, withdrawal protocols, the dangers of polypharmacy and the education of patients and their carers.

3 Who Will Be Involved in Training?

Trainers

It is essential to work in partnership with local counterparts to both ensure there is a good fit with needs, and for appropriate language/style and sustainability. This includes co-preparation and the delivery of training.

An example of where this has worked is the King's Somaliland partnership (see Chapters 14 and 15). This is an example of where training was delivered alongside local doctors. These doctors delivered the training alongside the international volunteers. Subsequently, those same local doctors delivered training independently.

Attendees

Even though you may have been given some information about the participants, it is good to find out as much as possible, so you can refine the training.

It can be difficult to find out who might be attending, what they already know and whether or not they speak English (or the languages you speak). But it is worth trying to find out! The host's selection of participants may bring together clinicians, administrators and sometimes other non-clinical people. Even within one professional group, there is the challenge of a group with mixed backgrounds, skill sets and language skills. In many countries there are hierarchies and social taboos that get played out in training. If doctors are with nurses, the latter may be quieter, and the former dominate. It takes good facilitation to get all to participate. One trainer recalls a training of all male doctors except for one female nurse. She did not say anything on day one. With careful facilitation and encouragement, by the end she was leading on volunteering to do role plays, able to give excellent insights and making the most out of the training.

It can be a challenge if you find out that there are military, government or opposition leaders in your group. Stepping aside from politics, the volunteer needs to be a diplomat as well as wearing all their other hats and work across differing groups with different views. You may hold your own views but remember to be a diplomat.

Stakeholders

If finding out who may be attending a training session, teaching event or workshop is challenging, finding out who matters to make the work sustainable is not only usually more difficult but possibly more important. Usually there are stakeholders in the local area: academics, government officials, traditional healers, district officials, businessmen, drug companies, NGOs and other international workers. Engaging as many potential allies as possible in discussions about the importance and value of the care of people with mental health problems is time well spent. For example, one team was invited to a thank you dinner after a two-week training event and found themselves in the midst of a heated discussion about who and which district would take forward a local pilot following the training sessions. The trainers regretted not engaging earlier with these key players to keep them all informed and involved. The future engagement of all stakeholders was essential to make the training sustainable.

If local dignitaries and stakeholders will be attending training sessions to welcome you or open the training events, find out who they are and how to address them.

Language and Translators

Direct translation may be necessary but sometimes asking for summaries from interpreters at intervals may be enough. Beware assurances that participants do all speak English. It is important to brief the translators and how you plan to work during the training; for example, whether it will be simultaneous translation or by allowing pauses. Remember that translators may be the only fully bilingual person you speak with, and they can give an invaluable insight into local culture.

Sometimes it is not entirely clear how accurate the translation has been, but a good translator can make the whole experience pleasant and easy for everyone. If there is no formal translator, you may be able to find someone in the audience who is sufficiently bilingual to assist. Or better still, co-facilitate with a local colleague or lecturer who can help with the language, include local issues and help facilitate the small group peer work.

The time spent translating can actually be a space for participants to think about what is being presented. New trainers who are more familiar with tight time frames at western conferences are inclined to rush into lots of information sharing and not leave sufficient time for digestion and discussion. Language difficulties can ruin a great programme and people may be too shy or embarrassed to tell you that they didn't understand. Even if your first language is English, your accent may make understanding difficult. Consider speaking more slowly than usual, be concise and keep checking if you have been understood.

4 When Can the Training Happen?

Timing

There will usually be a much more limited time available than trainers would like. Fitting sessions around other commitments is sometimes the only way participants can find enough time for training. Study leave and planned continuing professional development is new to many workers around the world. Getting time off clinical responsibilities can be challenging in low-resource settings. Taking time out of their clinical practice usually costs people money. Even if they are government employees and sent to training, there are still limits on days off work. This is where training and supervision needs to be seen as valuable by local providers as well as attendees. Sometimes attendees are paid a daily rate to attend, called *per diem* (per day). Sometimes there is a complex differential rate for per diems according to your professional role. If you do not know about per diems, you can be absolutely sure that those you are training are acutely aware. It is best to avoid being part of per diem distribution. Other incentives include certificates, training sessions with lunch included and opportunities to meet peers. There is rarely a budget for ongoing incentives and some organisations as a matter of principle do not pay per diems.

Finding a suitable time for trainers and trainees to meet for electronic training sessions can be quite challenging in global mental health settings. Asia is about six to seven hours ahead of GMT and the Americas are about five hours behind GMT.

Structuring a Timetable

The timetabling of training workshops is an art in itself. Usually, people have limited time for training events, and even if return visits or electronic follow-ups are planned, discernment is needed to agree on how best to use the time allocated. Decide what are the priorities. For example, is it better to spend more time on basic interviewing skills and concepts of mental illness, or assessment and management, human rights, drug and alcohol problems and other topics? Should record-keeping or safe prescribing be included? Should research, audit and getting published be mentioned or discussed? Teaching and facilitation skills?

Service development? There needs to be an active exercise in understanding what the participants want to discuss.

There is usually a need to allocate time for introductory and ending ceremonies, as well as the very important ritual of certificate giving and a group photograph. This needs consideration before people rush off on the final day with enough time to get home. Sometimes it is better to just accept that you cannot do everything that was planned and focus on what is important to the people gathered at this time, whilst keeping an eye on overall objectives and important areas like human rights in clinical practice. Helping people understand depression in depth, for example, may be more important than getting through the finer points of all the materials you have prepared. Remember the post-training evaluation and the need to leave time for 'what next'. Sustainable change is important. Discussions are needed about how participants can follow through with using their new skills clinically and get suitable ongoing support and supervision.

5 Where Will the Training Happen?

For face-to-face training, ensure there is a suitable venue. You may need to make sure you have the key to the training hall and bathroom facilities. Keep them on you or know who holds these. Double-check internet availability and how reliable it is. Be prepared by checking connection devices, flip charts, microphones, moveable chairs for interactive learning, handouts, evaluations, attendance lists, as well as translators' availability, style of working and languages spoken. Availability of suitable refreshments and lunch makes a difference to many people. See below for guidance on online training

6 How Will the Training Be Delivered?

Hosts may have particular views about desirable learning styles and training methods. For example, in Myanmar the monks and nuns at a workshop on mental health awareness said that they preferred formal lectures and plenty of time for reflection before discussions. They were, however, also curious about interactive training and said they also enjoyed the volunteers' efforts to combine different approaches.

Interactive Methods of Training

Lectures, workshops and discussion groups play an important role in teaching. At the same time, modern interactive methods may offer opportunities to provide participants with learning experiences that they will remember. Many people are inexperienced in interactive training methods but nonetheless welcome them. Historically, medicine has been taught in formal lecture formats, often without the opportunity for questions or clarification. It can be seen in some places as insulting to question a lecturer, as if he/she had not explained satisfactorily. Trainees and younger participants seem to welcome an interactive model. Older psychiatrists may not be quite so comfortable.

Planning plenty of interactive work also lessens the need to rely on language – 'don't tell me, show me'. Using diagrams, charts, images, demonstration role plays, quizzes and small group work help involve people and stimulate questions and discussion. In small group work, individual introductions can begin the formation of a working group and demonstrate the trainer's genuine interest in the thoughts, feelings and beliefs of participants. If there are language problems, using more small group work can help people learn from each other in their own languages. Small groups can be based around a presentation, a case discussion and include a role play. In larger groups, people can work in pairs and threes and the trainer can actually learn a lot by watching or 'eavesdropping' (with permission) on discussions. You can understand quite a lot about what is happening in a large group by careful observation. You will certainly see if people are just chatting, laughing or looking confused, and then you will be able to try to assist.

Delivering Training

The planning and checking have been done and now the participants arrive to sit and look at you. You take a deep breath and hope it will flow, despite realising that many things could go wrong. Containing your own anxiety can be a struggle. Day one is usually the hardest. After this period, you may find that you relax into a routine of following the programme. This will usually involve debriefing each evening and planning for the following day, whilst exploring the world around you, with new places to experience, foods to try and enjoying a sense of adventure.

Mostly, a well worked up project will go surprisingly well, especially if the participants are interested and not simply sent or told they must attend. Often something interesting happens, like extra people appearing or other curious professionals joining. For example, the trainers ask, 'who is that important looking person sitting up the back?' The host explains, 'Oh, he's a visiting professor who wants to know what you are doing.' Or a crowd arrives – 'Ah yes, those are our students.' See Table 8.4 for tips for training.

At the beginning of training, it is good practice to create ground rules that are generated by the participants, not you. Appoint a class lead so you can check what infraction of the rules actually means. In one example, there was someone who was always late. Later, the group learnt that she had to cross a dangerous frontline every morning to get to the venue. The class lead can guide you on how to manage the rules and understand the context of the participants. Lunch is always important and a time to get to know new colleagues and participants.

Table 8.4 Tips for training

- Be prepared but be flexible
- Set realistic goals that are agreed
- Go slow and speak slowly
- Less may be more – quality not quantity
- Get regular feedback with the help of the class lead
- Remember it is facilitating not teaching
- The experts are the participants
- Use local cases and local resources
- Use role play and videos
- Take care of participants – check refreshments, lunch, toilet breaks
- Behave professionally with courtesy, humanity and humility
- Self-care

Starting on the first day with a fun ice-breaking introductory exercise can help people relax and enjoy the day instead of settling in to be talked at for hours. One model that seems popular is giving a presentation such as a brief lecture, followed by a demonstration or video, and then group discussion or role play. You may need to use a presentation format such as PowerPoint, even though you need to be prepared to manage without it, in case of power failure or other unexpected dramas.

There are many PowerPoint presentations that support mhGAP[2] in many different languages, as an example. When using slide presentations, you will be wise to consider how best to adjust these to people whose first language is not English. Written English is usually better understood than spoken, especially where English educational material has been used in schools or colleges. For example, adjusting slides to include simple essential messages and key points is often helpful, and using slides to lead to exercises helps people understand what they are being asked to do; for example, 'Ms D brought her son to the nurse because he now wets the bed. Discuss what you would do.'

Word games and mnemonics can jog memories of complex subjects. Using the CATMAP (Table 8.5) can be particularly helpful as an adaptation of the key process of interaction with patients in WHO mhGAP.

Table 8.5 Basic principles of psychiatric skills – (mnemonic, CATMAP)

C for Communication
A for Assessment
T for Treatment
M for Mobilisation of social support
A for Attention to overall well-being
P for Protection of human rights

Confidence in setting up interactive training and making appropriate adjustments for culture may take some practice. However, it is worthwhile learning as participants in other countries report that they enjoy role play exercises and say that they have learnt a lot by practising in the clinician role as well as learning what matters to patients from being in their role.

Teaching techniques that are helpful include: case studies (see Box 8.2), paired discussions, small group and large group work, quizzes, videos (preferably with subtitles in appropriate languages), prepared digital teaching (again, ideally with subtitles, if needed), stories, posters, wall charts, and questions boxes (for the shy participants and difficult subjects like domestic violence). Alongside these interactive techniques, role play stands as the final arena of safe practising and experiential learning.

There is a skill in setting up a simple and successful role play. You may do well to work with an experienced partner or simply practise. Role plays work well by first demonstrating what happens, either using trainers as demonstrators, or a suitable video, and then asking people to gather in threes – one works as the clinician, another as the patient and the third person as observer. Exposing participants to trying it for the first time 'on stage' can be daunting and it usually works better by getting everyone to work in threes, either in their small groups or even in a large group. Table 8.6 suggests steps for basic role plays.

Table 8.6 Role play steps

Six steps of basic role play
1   Explain what will happen in this exercise, preferably by demonstrating a role play using trainers. Get participants in groups of three. Ask for volunteers to decide who will be the clinician, the patient and the observer
2   Get clinicians into role (e.g. if using WHO mhGAP, have the manual or phone app ready)
3   Get participants into role as patients, either using their own experience of the subject or a given role, asking them to use the first person (this is not a case discussion) and stay in role to help their colleague learn (appealing to altruism helps them stay in role at critical times)
4   Allocate times for role play action, announcing start and finish. Start with only 5 to10 minutes
5   De-role the patient. This is absolutely vital. Encourage them to stand up and shake off the role or say one way the real person is different to the role
6   Feedback is given to clinician from patient and observer, who has been told they have the most important job, which is true. Use only positive feedback, at least at the beginning of a training event

Other Training Essentials

Importance of Pre- and Post-Training Questionnaires

It may be appropriate to do a pre-training assessment of trainees on the first morning to compare with a post-training repeated evaluation afterwards to check what changes have been made. A good way to check the knowledge, skills and attitude of a group can be a brief questionnaire. Usually there is limited time to do a full assessment of the current knowledge of attendees. A brief form, taking 15–20 minutes, with true/false questions and some clinical scenarios, coupled with a request to write a case study about someone with possible mental illness, gives trainers a reasonably good idea about participants' concerns as well as their English language proficiency and knowledge about mental health.

It is helpful for questionnaires to be anonymised unless people add their names voluntarily. These can be coded with an identifier that can be reidentified at the end of training evaluation. It is possible to create bespoke pre- and post-evaluations or use one that is already devised such as the mhGAP pre- and post-test. The participants need to know that this is a voluntary assessment for guiding the training and not an exam for them. Reassure them that the results will be anonymised and confidential. Written permission would be needed for any formal research, and this would take time, as participants may be unfamiliar with research protocols and complex legal language. It can also create an atmosphere of confusion and concern about what the trainers are doing. As such, any research needs to be handled with care and adequate planning, including co-development.

Case Studies
Case studies can show gender and social issues, like polygamy and forced marriage, that are important for trainers from outside to understand. Usually, participants highlight adult mental health conditions, often with more female than male patients. Child and adolescent conditions may be missed, and dementia not mentioned or equated with old age. Intellectual disability is often rarely mentioned or only gets briefly mentioned as

a condition in children. It is surprising how similar clinical problems are around the world. In secondary care there is the usual focus on psychosis and substance use disorders. In primary care, in many countries, there are concerns in areas of somatisation, anxiety disorders, substance misuse and epilepsy. Depression can often be 'hidden' by physical complaints. What may be less familiar to volunteers from the UK may be conversion disorders and pseudo-seizures. In Nepal, the trainers were told that cases of trance and possessions states are often seen. Here they listened to how the hosts managed such conditions. Substance abuse varies – in Somalia Qat/khat is used frequently. In the Middle East, tramadol is often used, and in Ukraine it is alcohol misuse.

In one training, 60% of case studies collected on day one contained concerns about drug and alcohol use and so it was necessary to rearrange the programme on the first evening, to accommodate this. The case studies can also be useful for role plays, as well as discussion points.

Online Training

Since the Covid-19 outbreak, much training has moved online. This poses challenges as trainers continue to learn the skills of online facilitation and learn to stretch the limits and use creative solutions. The main challenge is to engage with participants and provide an interactive platform of learning. Table 8.7 offers tips for online training.

Online training can vary in how it is delivered. Options include:

- Contemporaneous online training
- Synchronous and asynchronous training
- Online web-based self-directed learning

Table 8.7 Tips for online training

- Be well-prepared
- Share background documents beforehand
- Have clear ground rules
- Have an attendance list for every session
- Ensure everyone has their video on as much as possible
- Use chat box creatively
- Use break-out rooms for small group work and for peer learning
- Use demonstration role plays and role plays with participants
- Have a full list of participants ready and call out names for questions
- Use different tools including videos
- Have lots of small breaks
- Make use of facial expression and body language
- Use lots or repetition and checking people have understood
- Use more true and false questions as tools of engagement
- Have asummary at the end of the day and recap next morning
- Use interpreters – try to ignore their presence and speak directly to participants
- Can have supplementary individual Zoom meetings to do evaluations at the end of the training

Contemporaneous Online Training

This is probably the easiest as it can mimic face-to-face training except it is on an online platform. There can be one or multiple facilitators. Translation can be easily accommodated. This is usually with each participant online on their own screen. However, occasionally participants may be together in one room with a large screen. The chat function can be extremely useful as well as online polls and the liberal use of break-out rooms. Challenges to this format are engagement. Participants may leave their cameras off, and this makes it very difficult to engage with them. Sometimes bandwidth may make leaving the camera off preferable. This is probably the biggest obstacle to training. The facilitator should have all the names of participants ready and call out names. When their names are called out, they can be invited to speak, answer questions and turn on the camera at that time. Another technique is to ask a selection of people to turn their camera on to ease training. To facilitate peer learning, and cultural and linguistic comfort, the participants can be readily encouraged to perform exercises in pairs if in one room and in small break-out rooms. Participants appreciate the opportunity to speak in their own language. The facilitators can drop in on each room to check progress. Training like this needs to be small to enable effective learning of knowledge and skills, for example 20 to 30. Larger groups can be less effective but more conducive to a traditional lecture format. As an example, the author has conducted a recent online training with a group who were in one room. There was simultaneous translation in Russian. The names of the participants were called out for questions and to organise tasks. The participants were invited to do a lot of paired activities at their table which they could do in their own language. This was complemented by demonstration role plays by the facilitators. The chat function allowed multiple choice and true and false questions. In another training, individual assessments on Zoom were used to check on skills acquisition through role play with the facilitator.

Synchronous and Asynchronous Training

Here there can be a mixture of self-directed learning using a selection of web-based resources. As an example, there can be a core video with lecture format complemented by resources of academic papers, quizzes and first-person patient stories on podcast or video. There is a component that is live, with a shared webinar format. For example, in an 18-country teaching programme, there was a schedule of live lectures and teaching as well as other self-directed resources for people to explore. In addition to this, there was homework. One of the other components was a forum for online questions and answers. There was a clear timetable that participants had to move through in order to achieve a certificate of completion.

Online Web-Based Self-Directed Learning

This is asynchronous learning as self-directed by participants at their own pace. In reality there can be a combination of all of these to make an effective training. For example, there can be a hybrid training that is face to face with one of the facilitators joining online.

There are other online functions that are very helpful, such as supervision. For example, one of the authors was able to supervise health workers in South Sudan, Northeast Syria and refugee camps in Africa, when travel was not possible. For supervision, the platform can be Skype, Zoom, WhatsApp or whatever works best for participants. Internet problems can be a challenge and multiple different platforms may be needed. WhatsApp is currently ubiquitous and can be a very easy vehicle for supervision.

The Future of Training

Online facilities have transformed our ability to work globally for both training and other development activities. Digital meetings, webinars and training sessions can be organised quickly and successfully. This will undoubtedly develop and hopefully open up closer working partnerships in global mental health by more regular communications and the sharing of ideas, information and materials.

Electronic connectivity will also help with the really big challenge of ongoing supervision and sustainability. Efforts to find a way to establish ongoing contact and support are vital. The feedback from short training (e.g. two weeks intensive) is usually good immediately post-event, but what about the future? Ongoing support and supervision for bedding down new clinical practices into day-to-day work can be difficult to organise and maintain. A new innovation is the EQUIP platform (Ensuring Quality in Psychological Support)[19].

There is a saying that one-off short training is 'entertainment only' and that many months of interactive support is needed to really make improvements in clinical practice. Planning for ongoing learning needs to be built into the programme, even before leaving the UK. Research into what might work best for ongoing support is much needed.

Training Elements Checklist

Table 8.8 An outline of elements to consider when delivering training to mitigate some of the challenges

Training delivery elements checklist
Preparation meeting with hosts to agree objectives
Training resources: materials, microphones, internet, etc.
Meet with interpreters
Attendance list including titles, affiliations and contact (e-mail/telephone)
Introductions and opening ceremony
Ground rules and group representative
Pre- and post-test evaluations
Timetabling and agreement to keep to time
Refreshments, lunch and other breaks
Certificates and closing ceremony
Plan for follow up
Team/host meeting to review training
Summary report

Conclusion

Attention to delivery of training with careful discussions between host and volunteers as to the 'Why, What, Who, When, Where and How', plus a dash of flexibility can provide a satisfying experience for both host and volunteers who can learn a great deal from the experience, and each other.

The importance of psychological as well as pharmacological treatments is becoming a key area in global mental health. Training using interactive methods helps practitioners learn to engage with training and practise new skills.

The incorporation of online learning into global mental health means changes, some of which will be welcome – quicker communication, sending reading and training modules ahead of possible face-to-face meetings, easy access to ongoing conversations, coupled with less travel and a greener footprint – is balanced by the loss of the possibility of enjoyable social time with new colleagues and less cultural experiences.

References

1. World Health Organization. mhGAP intervention guide for mental, neurological and substance use disorders in non-specialized health settings: mental health Gap Action Programme (mhGAP), version 2.0 ed. Geneva: World Health Organization; 2016.

2. World Health Organization. mhGAP humanitarian intervention guide (mhGAP-HIG): clinical management of mental, neurological and substance use conditions in humanitarian emergencies. World Health Organization; 2015.

3. World Health Organization. Psychological first aid: guide for field workers. World Health Organization; 2011.

4. Epping-Jordan JE, Harris R, Brown FL et al. Self-Help Plus (SH+): a new WHO stress management package. World Psychiatry. 2016;15(3):295.

5. World Health Organization. Problem Management Plus (PM+): individual psychological help for adults impaired by distress in communities exposed to adversity. World Health Organization; 2016.

6. World Health Organization. Thinking healthy: a manual for psychosocial management of perinatal depression, WHO generic field-trial, version 1.0. World Health Organization; 2015. Report No.: 9754004110.

7. World Health Organization. Group interpersonal therapy (IPT) for depression. World Health Organization; 2016.

8. World Health Organization. Doing what matters in times of stress: an illustrated guide; 2020.

9. World Health Organization. Building back better: sustainable mental health care after emergencies. World Health Organization; 2013.

10. World Psychiatric Association. Education Portal. www.wpanet.org/education-portal.

11. Scotland-Malawi Mental Health Education Project. 2020. www.smmhep.org.uk/sites/default/files/eMalawi Quick Guide to Mental Health v1 (1).pdf.

12. Mental Health and Psychosocial Support Network. Mental health and psychosocial Support. https://app.mhpss.net.

13. Mental Health Innovation Network M. www.mhinnovation.net.

14. World Health Organization. WHO Quality Rights tool kit: assessing and improving quality and human rights in mental health and social care facilities. World Health Organization; 2012.

15. Patel V, Hanlon C. Where There Is No Psychiatrist: A Mental Health Care Manual. 2nd ed. Cambridge: Royal College of Psychiatrists; 2018.

16. Eapen V, Graham P, Srinath S. Where there is no child psychiatrist: a mental

healthcare manual. RCPsych publications; 2012.

17. World Health Organization. Mental health atlas 2017. Geneva: World Health Organization; 2018. https://apps.who.int/iris/handle/10665/272735.

18. World Health Organization. World Health Organization assessment instrument for mental health systems-WHO-AIMS, version 2.2. World Health Organization; 2005.

19. Ensuring Quality in Psychological Support. www.who.int/teams/mental-health-and-substance-use/treatment-care/equip-ensuring-quality-in-psychological-support.

Psychological Techniques Toolkit

Bradley Hillier, Peter Hughes and Sophie Thomson

Introduction

Making diagnoses and understanding the appropriate use of medication in treating mental disorders is just one part of mental health care. The other part is psychosocial treatments. In global volunteering it is important to be skilled in the principles and use of these psychological treatments as well as medication. Some aspects of medication are included here as there is so much interplay of psychosocial and prescribing.

In global mental health, using the term Mental Health and Psychosocial Support (MHPSS) reminds us of the importance of both aspects of treatment. The *WHO mhGAP Intervention Guide v 2.0*[1] also reminds us of this key message in treating patients and their families.

Through the course of various volunteering projects including delivering teaching of the WHO mhGAP with the Royal College of Psychiatrists' Volunteering and International Psychiatry Special Interest Group (VIPSIG)[2], a new 'Toolkit' has been developed. This now forms a core part of training in mental health, particularly for frontline clinicians. This can equip health care workers with practical, easily learnt and remembered skills in psychosocial support. Experience and feedback suggest that these practical skills are very helpful. Health workers say that they have learnt something that they can use in their everyday clinical practice.

The toolkit is used in the context of the WHO mhGAP[1]. In the chapter called Essential Care and Practice, this manual lays down the foundation principles of good mental health care practice. The mhGAP Humanitarian version has a similar chapter called General Principles of Care[3]. The elements in these chapters emphasise:

- Communication
- Respect and dignity
- Assessing mental, physical and social health
- Managing mental, physical and social health

Psychosocial treatments specifically mentioned include:

- Psycho-education
- Reducing stress and strengthening social support
- Promoting functioning in daily activities
- 'Formal' psychological treatments, where available

Included in these topics are human rights, ethical principles, challenging stigma and attending to self-care, and all have a bearing on psychosocial skills. Medication may be needed but, if so, only after psychosocial treatments have been explored. Medication is not always necessary.

Following these principles can mean changes in practice as simple as making sure practitioners have the opportunity to see a patient alone in a clinic, thereby preserving confidentiality. In many countries the patient will arrive with their immediate and even extended family and being able to speak freely is not possible. Having the opportunity for a confidential discussion can transform the experience for both clinician and patient.

Assessment Screening Tool for Mental Illness

Another tool that can be helpful is 'The Golden Questions' taken from 'Where There is No Psychiatrist'[4] (Table 9.1). The Golden Questions are particularly useful in primary care. They can be a useful screen for mental illness and save a lot of time.

The health worker should also check if children, disabled people and carers have any mental health problems as these are often missed.

Table 9.1 The Golden Questions

1. Do you have any problems **sleeping** at night?
2. Have you been feeling as if you have **lost interest** in your usual activities?
3. Have you been feeling **sad** or unhappy recently?
4. Have you been feeling **scared** or frightened of anything?
5. Have you been worried about **taking drugs or too much alcohol** recently?
6. How much money and time have you been spending on **drugs** or alcohol recently?

Additional useful questions
  - What worries does your family have about you?
  - Have you experienced economic problems?
  - Have you any problems at home?

The VIPSIG Toolkit

The authors have developed a pictorial image of a person to make an easily remembered toolkit of simple psychological skills for all health workers to employ.

In a training session, individual psychosocial techniques can be explained, demonstrated and practised and added to a wall chart. Each participant also is invited to make their own diagram to suit their practice. As an example, in Figure 9.1 the parts of the body are used symbolically to remind health workers about key skills. The different techniques are placed at different parts of the body as an aide memoire and symbolic meaning. Table 9.2 details the skills illustrated in Figure 9.1 and links each skill to appropriate mental health conditions. Each of the 13 skills are then explained in detail.

Mental state examination is included as this is part of the dynamic interaction between health worker and patient. It reflects rapport building, good communication skills and psychiatric/psychosocial formulation.

Hopefully practitioners will find these psychological skills, techniques and approaches useful both in primary and secondary care. The characteristics of these psychosocial 'tools' are as follows:

  - relevant and applicable to a range of mental health problems seen in primary and secondary care
  - simple to teach
  - simple to learn and use
  - zero (or minimal) financial cost

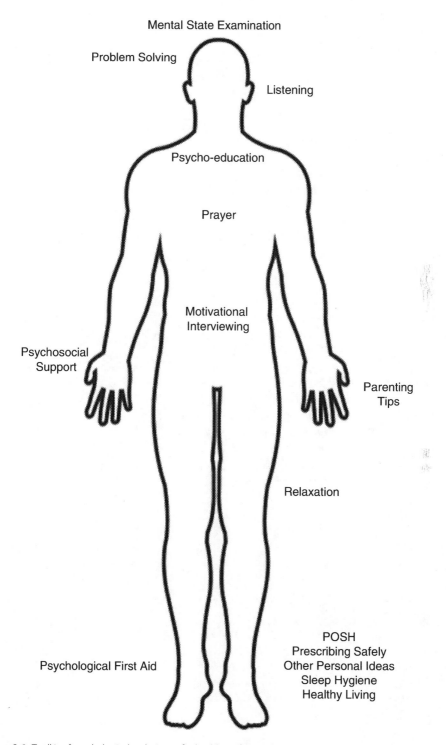

Mental State Examination

Problem Solving

Listening

Psycho-education

Prayer

Motivational
Interviewing

Psychosocial
Support

Parenting
Tips

Relaxation

POSH
Prescribing Safely
Other Personal Ideas
Sleep Hygiene
Healthy Living

Psychological First Aid

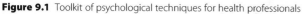

Figure 9.1 Toolkit of psychological techniques for health professionals

Table 9.2 Toolkit of simple psychological techniques for health professionals and linked mental health conditions

Skill	Summary of skill	Mental health conditions
1. Psycho-education	Communication of important and relevant information	All
2. Listening	Active listening is a key skill in ensuring people feel heard and understood	All
3. Psychosocial support	Uses the 'Hand Technique' to remind people about supportive contacts, therapeutic activities and personal sayings that are helpful in difficult times	All
4. Problem-solving	Problem-solving involves exploring options to solve problems, and access available resources	All, but particularly in depression, dementia, stress, child and adolescent problems and substance misuse-related problems
5. Parenting skills	Gives simple advice that clinicians can use to help parents manage family difficulties	Child and adolescent problems
6. Psychological first aid (PFA)	PFA skills are about grounding and attention to basic needs during acutely stressful times	Stress-related and emergency situations
7. Prescribing safely	Safe and appropriate prescribing, based on up-to-date evidence and research	All
8. Relaxation techniques	Simple skills including breathing techniques and muscle relaxation	Particularly helpful with anxiety disorders
9. Sleep hygiene	Useful for many mental health conditions	All
10. Motivational interviewing	Useful for changing behaviour, especially drug and alcohol misuse	Substance misuse problems and broader applicability to many health conditions
11. Mental state examination	Can be learnt in primary care	All
12. Prayer/spiritual beliefs	Spiritual beliefs and prayer life need attention as they are very important to many people.	All
13. Attention to overall well-being	Healthy living advice e.g. alcohol and drug use, food, tobacco	All

Psychological Techniques in the Toolkit

1 Psycho-education

This is always relevant for any mental health difficulty. Simple information provided by health workers can be reassuring, reduce stigma and promote recovery. Psycho-education involves providing information about mental health conditions to the person and their family, including what the condition is, its expected course and outcome, available treatments, duration of treatment and expected benefits, as well as potential side effects of any medication, if needed.

A useful questions to ask here is '*what do you think caused this problem?*' This may reveal if there are any beliefs that might be relevant. For example, the person may believe that their problem is spiritual, caused by witchcraft or they are convinced it is a purely physical problem.

People may have assumptions in attending a health worker. People may expect to receive medication or have investigations. Psycho-education is an opportunity to sensitively deal with these assumptions. Many prescriptions are not appropriate, such as unnecessary vitamins, incorrect doses of psychotropics and polypharmacy. A simple explanation of mental health problems can be an alternative to inappropriate prescribing.

It is likely that in many countries the person will have gone to see a traditional or religious healer first. Using a non-judgmental approach and explaining that this is acceptable and that it may well complement seeing a health worker can be helpful. Leaflets on the mental health conditions may also be useful, if appropriate and available. These can be pictorial for non-literate people.

For volunteers it may be difficult to fully understand how to frame messages of psycho-education for a particular culture. A particular issue can be local spiritual beliefs. Global partners and hosts will be able to develop the appropriate psycho-education message – the mhGAP-IG psycho-education sections are a good starting point.

2 Listening Skills

Basic listening skills can be readily taught and are especially useful for people who have little opportunity to learn more complex skills. Training can place a significant emphasis on the importance of active and attentive listening through both demonstration role play, small group work, discussion and practice. Positive feedback is encouraged within role plays to support development of confidence. Repeated practice of good listening is encouraged when new skills are added.

As a training tool it can be useful to demonstrate a good and a bad communication role play. A simple exercise that participants can do to demonstrate the skill of attentive listening is to work in a pair where one person is the 'listener' and they listen to the other person speak for a defined time, such as two or three minutes, about an aspect of themselves or their lives, without interrupting or taking notes. They then repeat back what they have heard the other person say about themselves and then carry out the exercise in the opposite direction. Reflection within the pair about how this style of attentive listening with 'ears, eyes and heart' contrasts with the usual way we listen, but possibly don't hear, and allows for an appreciation of the qualitative difference highlighted during the exercise. Through modelling of listening skills and this experiential practice, the health worker can learn to replicate good listening in their own consultations with patients.

It is important to remind health workers to include children, people with intellectual disability and people with dementia in their listening. These people may communicate differently but they need to be heard too.

3 Psychosocial Support and the 'Hand Technique'

The reduction of stress and getting support when people are feeling vulnerable is a key part of managing most mental health conditions. Strengthening personal and social resources is an important skill for volunteers to learn.

The word 'psychosocial' refers to the inter-relationship between the psychological and social worlds experienced by an individual. For the purpose of providing a simple and easy aide memoire for use in primary care settings the 'Hand Technique' can be taught. This relies on the principle that people can use their hand and can link parts of their hand such as the fingers or lines with people, activities and sayings that provide them with support.

Using the Hand Technique in its three parts consists of:

First, for each finger of the person's hand, prompt them to remember a person to whom the patient could turn for support (including but not limited to family members, and may even be people who are not physically present). Prompt by asking about friends, neighbours, extended family, local organisations, community and religious leaders to whom they could turn. This is an example of social mobilisation. Examples include: fingers representing family members, friends old and new, distant or even deceased relatives, priest or sheikh, MSF, other organisations. It is important that the person creates their own examples for their potential support.

Second, for the two lines across the hand, ask people to recall or identify two activities that are helpful (or used to be comforting or soothing) to that individual. This is an example of behavioural activation. People need to generate their own personal examples to be most effective. Typical examples are listening to music, playing football, talking to friends, swimming, cooking and walks in nature. Unhelpful activities can be discussed such as alcohol, smoking and other substances which might make problems worse. Third, for the two creases across the wrist, reflect or identify two sayings, phrases or affirmations that are personally meaningful. These can take some thinking about, but again should be self-generated for the best effect. Examples we have seen are: '*I am never alone, there is always someone to speak to*', '*last time something like this happened I coped and overcame the problem*', '*All is in divine order*' and '*just put one foot in front of the other*'.

A simple diagram could be provided in the health worker's clinic or they could use the hand of their patient to demonstrate, if culturally appropriate (see Figure 9.2).

The Hand Technique is particularly useful for children but is helpful for all ages. General practitioners here in the UK have given feedback on how useful the Hand Technique can be for many conditions and situations.

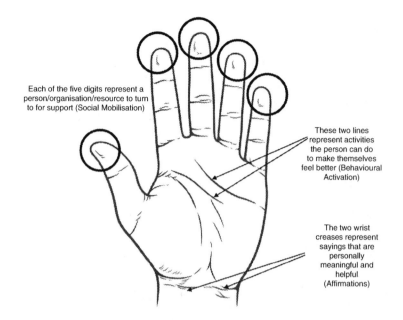

Each of the five digits represent a person/organisation/resource to turn to for support (Social Mobilisation)

These two lines represent activities the person can do to make themselves feel better (Behavioural Activation)

The two wrist creases represent sayings that are personally meaningful and helpful (Affirmations)

Figure 9.2 Hand technique

4 Simple Problem-Solving Skills

Many mental health problems are rooted in, or compounded by, problems in a person's life. Everyday problems can lead to substance use, suicidal feelings, depression, somatic symptoms, conversion disorder and other problems. Dealing with problems is important and the skill is in helping the person solve their own problems. Often there are many problems for which there is no easy solution, for example grinding poverty, injustice, violence. The technique works best by finding small problems that are amenable to change.

Problem-solving can help people understand that they do have resources to improve their lives, albeit in small ways, and hence it can be empowering.

Often people will find it difficult to separate out individual problems and say they have numerous or too many to count. On average there are about five or six. Economic and relationship problems are almost always at the top, along with marital concerns, worries about children and even mothers-in-law. Asking what makes the mental health symptom worse or better can help focus on what the relevant problems might be, for example, *'my headache is worse when I have a fight with my husband, and it is better when I spend time with my children.'* Health workers usually know about local resources that may be able to help discussions about possible solutions.

The WHO has produced the 'Problem Management Plus' (PM+) manual[5] which comprehensively describes a very useful empowering method of assisting adults in communities exposed to adversity to find their own best solutions to specific challenges. Delivery of this training is a specific course in itself and suitable for situations where there is a more permanent presence of field workers working in mental health organisations.

A shortened 'bedside' version can be used and taught in busy clinical practice for health practitioners using key principles with a five-stage method. These are shown in Table 9.3, with an illustrated examples in Table 9.4.

Table 9.3 Principles of problem-solving

- Ask what the main problems are
- Define more carefully exactly what is the most important problem that might be amenable to change
- Help the person generate options, ensuring the person explores their own their ideas, with as little prompting as possible
- Decide on one option and work together to set up a plan for action
- Arrange follow-up to celebrate success and/or make another plan

Table 9.4 Example of problem-solving

Example of problem-solving – patient (P) and health worker (HW)

HW: Can you tell me what are the stresses/problems you have at the moment?

P: I have so many I can't even think. It is all too much.

HW: Tell me what is the biggest problem or what would you like to talk about today?

P: I have no money, my husband has no job, I have no job. I can't afford to buy shoes for my children to go to school. I am so ashamed.

HW: That's a lot and sounds difficult. You have given me five problems.
What is the most important problem right now?

P: The biggest problem now is getting shoes for my children.

HW: What are your thoughts on what might be possible solutions?

P: I don't know. I have no money.

HW: Is there anyone who can help you?

P: I could speak to my sister maybe?

HW: That's a good idea. Is it possible she will help you?

P: I will go to my sister and see if she can help me. Maybe she will lend me enough to go to the charity shop downtown and buy shoes. It's been good just to talk and be listened to. That makes me feel better.

HW: That's good and next time we can see how you are feeling and if you want to explore other problems. Do you have any questions?

P: No, that has helped me. Goodbye.

A training example that is often used is the problem of an elderly relative with dementia who wanders and places themselves in vulnerable situations. Options generated by the patient and family can typically include the relative living with a family member, taking the person out regularly at fixed times and asking neighbours for support.

The patient almost always has a creative solution if they are encouraged and well supported. If not, the health worker has done a good job by listening non-judgmentally.

5 Parenting Skills and Star Chart

Problems with children and adolescents are reported as a major challenge for many families, and health workers can often feel unskilled in offering advice. Key universal points on how to improve behaviour in the chapter on Childhood Conditions in mhGAP Intervention Guide can be easily taught (see Table 9.5). Collecting ideas about good parenting in the local area or country can be compared with WHO mhGAP suggestions. Usually there is considerable agreement and a good discussion by a training group ensues.

Physical punishment is often a subject of debate as it can be considered normal and even advisable in some places. This needs to be dealt with non-judgmentally. One of the main messages is to show your child that you love them and look at their strengths.

Demonstration role plays followed by practice role plays, whereby health practitioners practise themselves, helps them to feel much more confident in trying to offer evidence-based advice and not use medication.

There is almost no case (apart from epilepsy) when medication is the only appropriate and available treatment for children. Unfortunately, children with hyperactivity or other problems can sometimes be prescribed strong medication including antipsychotic drugs. Health practitioners teaching key family members basic parenting skills can make this less likely to continue.

A skill that is very powerful and easily implemented is the use of the reward or star chart to support changing problematic behaviours. This has a strong evidence base (e.g. in nocturnal enuresis – bed-wetting[6]). An example of the bedwetting scenario is provided in Table 9.6. Many health workers in low- and middle-income countries (LMICs) are not familiar with the principles behind this intervention of the pairing of positive or desired behaviours with a reward.

Table 9.5 Parenting skills

- Give loving attention, including playing with the child
- Be consistent and clear about the rules with simple instructions
- Give daily tasks that match ability and offer praise
- Praise good behaviour and give no reward when behaviour is problematic
- Find ways to avoid severe confrontations
- Make punishment mild and infrequent
- Do not use threats or physical punishment. It can make behaviour worse
- Speak to a child when feeling calm, not when angry
- Help the child feel as safe and secure as possible even when it may not be safe or secure
- Encourage age-appropriate play
- Attend to their basic needs
- Ensure education
- Treat all children equally – boys and girls

Table 9.6 Bedwetting scenario – mother (M) and health worker (HW)

M: My son is 9 years old, and he is bed-wetting. He is very bad, and I beat him. Can you give him strong medicines please?

HW: Where is your son now?

M: He is at school.

HW: Did beating him help?

M: No, it made him worse.

HW: Maybe we can try something different?

M: OK, as it is very stressful.

HW: Has he any physical health problems? Was he dry before?

M: No problems. He was dry and now wet since he went to new school. He has some problems at school.

HW: I see. I think we need to look at the problems at school as well and I need to do a physical examination. But now I suggest we do this technique called the star chart. Bring him in next time so I can show him as well. Can I please check to see if you can manage to read the chart ok?

M: I can read numbers and days of the week.

HW: OK, this is simple. I will give you these calendars for a few months. Each day in the calendar represents a night – a dry night is a tick or a little star and praise him. A wet night is left blank. Do this with him. If he gets three ticks, you can reward him. Maybe by doing something with him he likes. For a wet night just ignore and don't punish. After a month he is likely to improve. I will see you then to check again. Have you any questions?

M: No, that is clear. Next time maybe I can also see what I can do about his

HW: Yes, the school problems may be making this problem worse, but we can work on both at same time.

6 Psychological First Aid (PFA)

The WHO manual 'Psychological First Aid: Guide for Field Workers'[7] makes clear that PFA can and should be learnt by as many people as possible. Any and all professionals involved in frontline care can learn this and feel confident about what to do in acutely stressful situations. It is useful for emergencies, large and small, from mass disasters to individual traumatic situations involving interpersonal violence. In delivering training, this skill is linked with acute stress situations in particular and can be combined with communication skills training. This helps the way in which rapport can be established with traumatised patients. In practical terms, demonstration role plays using bad and good clinical examples are particularly effective.

PFA involves ensuring and supporting the essential human needs of feeling as safe as possible, with basic warmth, drinks and shelter, and contact with family and important others. The person needs to be listened to and not left alone, as well as being offered appropriate medical care. The person is not expected to discuss what happened unless they want to do so. It is important to emphasise that critical incident debriefing is not recommended[1]. Formerly, it was believed that it was necessary to talk about a stressful event, regardless of whether one wanted to or not. It is now known that making someone talk about something that they do not feel ready to talk about can be traumatising in its own way rather than helpful. See Table 9.7 for an illustrated example of PFA.

Table 9.7 Example case of using Psychological First Aid (PFA) – patient (P) and health worker (HW)

A 20-year-old woman comes into a health clinic soon after an emergency. She says she has been raped.

P: It is really hard for me to come here and say what has happened.

HW: I can see you are really upset. Are you OK to talk to me, or would you prefer to see a female worker?

P: I am OK to speak to you. I have been raped but I can't bring myself to speak about it.

HW: That is OK. Are you safe now? Do you have a place to stay that is safe? Have you money for food and people who can help you? Also do you want me to help you get to the hospital to be examined? I can help you talk to the police if you want me to help with that.
　　Have you had anything to eat today or drink? Let me get you something.

P: Thank you. I don't want to go to the police. I don't want to talk about it.
　　I don't have a place to live now since the earthquake.

HW: OK, let me make a call to see where there is a safe place to stay and see if we can get you some money to help you. If you want to talk about what happened, then we can do that when you feel ok to do so. Are you managing to look after yourself overall? Do you think you are coping enough to look after yourself? Can I call someone in your family to help you?

P: I don't have any phone credit. Could you phone my sister for me as I can probably stay with her safely?

HW: OK, and then can I organise to see you tomorrow and check how you are or telephone you.

P: Thanks.

7 Prescribing Safely and Appropriately

Part of good psychosocial care is education about medication. Safe prescribing is very much part of the skills needed in good clinical practice. This includes ensuring that the patient and their families understand their medication.

Although not strictly a psychosocial skill, education about medication and safe prescribing is very much part of the skills in good practice and rational prescribing. It demands good psychosocial skills. WHO mhGAP details the importance of safe prescribing with appropriate drug, dose, duration and side effects, and lists a number of the core medications, their use and side effect profile, and where there is a need for specialist monitoring. 'Start low' (doses) and 'go slow' (increase slowly) is the usual 'mantra'. It is important that the decision about taking a medicine is the patient's and theirs alone, supported by good information. The days of doctors telling the patient what to do unquestioningly and unchallengingly are hopefully gone. Good communication and information about any medicine are essential.

It is helpful to understand in advance the main psychotropic medications which may be available and used in the country, and information about this can be obtained from the WHO, or at a more local level from health workers themselves. Common errors can be too high a dose of antipsychotics and too low a dose of antidepressants.

The aim is to ensure that key messages of polypharmacy and serious side effects of psychotropic medications are covered as well as dependency issues for certain medication groups, and special situations such as pregnancy and high-risk self-harm situations. Knowledge of local street drugs and their effects can also inform important discussions.

It is useful to discuss possible unintentional dangerous prescribing occurring. One example was finding that a psychotropic medication (Clozapine) was being prescribed in primary care as night sedation after a recent drug company visit.

A significant aspect of this toolkit item practised during training sessions is a discussion regarding the motivations and ethics of prescribing medications that are known to be ineffective (often vitamins). In clinical practice, discussion and negotiation about such treatments could be coupled with one of the other non-pharmacological psychosocial 'toolkit' interventions (as is demonstrated in some of the International Medical Corps' mhGAP training videos[8]).

Sometimes support is needed to identify and foster relationships with local psychiatric services, where health care workers can get advice, information and support.

8 Relaxation Techniques

The usefulness of relaxation methods for anxiety in various forms is now well-accepted. Techniques include simple breathing routines, progressive muscle relaxations and meditation. Through experiential learning, the health workers are shown and then practise a method that suits them and that they can teach to patients. For example, trainers can use an online video or engage health workers to share practices that they may already use for themselves or their patients. Practice in role plays helps to make this possible. In some countries which have a tradition of meditation, it is possible to relate these techniques to the practice of mindfulness and the potential benefits for mental health problems[9].

Each volunteer should ideally be confident in at least two different breathing techniques. One could be deep muscle relaxation and the other could be basic 'bedside' breathing exercises (see Table 9.8). It is important to practise these techniques, which can be used to help insomnia, stress and somatic pain and generalised anxiety.

Table 9.8 Example breathing exercise

Step 1 Sit comfortably or lie down in a quiet place
Step 2 Close your eyes
Step 3 Concentrate on your breathing
Step 4 Normal breath through nose for count of three – inhale
Step 5 Normal breath out through mouth for count of four – exhale
Step 6 Repeat for 10 minutes – practise so you can use it day to day

9 Sleep Hygiene

It is well-established that many mental health conditions affect sleep, and a knowledge of sleep hygiene may help reduce, or be used in combination with, the use of medication[10]. Straightforward advice such as that in Table 9.9 can be provided to patients. It is important to recognise the limits and application of such sleep hygiene techniques when there is potentially precarious or overcrowded accommodation.

Table 9.9 Sleep hygiene techniques

- Avoid caffeine and alcohol late in the day
- Avoid working, texting, etc. in bed. Bed is for sleep
- Avoid taking naps, especially late in the day
- Go to sleep and wake up at the same times each day
- Keep the bedroom relaxing, dark and at a comfortable temperature
- Set aside time to relax and get into a bedtime routine

10 Motivational Interviewing and the Cycle of Change

The basic principles and simplified application of motivational interviewing can be taught to all clinicians.

The WHO manual 'Alcohol, Smoking and Substance Involvement Screening Test (ASSIST)'[11] and associated programme publications describe an in-depth strategy and approach to the assessment and management of substance misuse issues, including motivational interviewing techniques for health workers, although this requires detailed training in itself.

In primary care settings, it can be valuable to outline the principles of motivational interviewing not simply as a technique to use in substance use disorders, but as a broader method to approach and facilitate changes in behaviour using the model proposed by Proschka and diClemente[12], as shown in Figure 9.3. A basic understanding of the cycle of change can equip the health worker with a valuable tool to approach traditional doctor-patient interactions regarding not only substance use disorder, but various health conditions in an alternative manner to the paternalistic style of telling people what to do. It also provides an alternative framework to pharmacologically focused styles of communication and assists in the development of listening skills. It helps health care workers to be realistic about what might be possible and not to be too discouraged by repeated relapses from abstinence or repeated unhelpful behaviours.

The cycle of change can be explained to patients and is a core aspect of individuals understanding where they are in their own recovery from substance use. There are also mnemonics which can be used to outline the principles and practice of motivational interviewing approaches. A popular plan is listed in Table 9.10 using mnemonics[13].

Using techniques like these, health workers can help their patients to link their own motivations to changing their behaviour/substance use, which is much more effective than telling people what to do and appearing judgmental.

Motivational interviewing also includes discussing the benefits and disadvantages of continuing to abuse alcohol and/or substances and, once again, this assists people to make their own decisions without being told what to do by someone else. This is demonstrated in the example in Table 9.11.

Table 9.10 Principles of motivational interview mnemonics – OARS

Open questions: Using these allows the patient to tell their story

Affirmations: Sincere acknowledgement of the patient's hard work and efforts

Reflective Listening: Reflecting back what the patient has said, demonstrating a genuine desire to understand them

Summarising: 3–4 sentences summarising what has been said, and checking that patient and clinician are on the same page

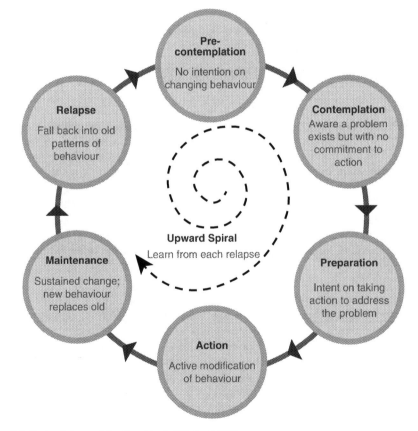

Figure 9.3 Cycle of change (after Proschka & diClemente[12])

Table 9.11 Motivational interviewing, simplified version – health worker (HW) and patient (P)

HW: Good morning. Thank you for coming to see me. I believe your wife has asked you to come along to see me today.

P: Yes, sir. She is unhappy about how much I drink, and we quarrel a lot. I came here to stop her fighting with me.

HW: OK. Can we talk about your drinking? Firstly – what are the good things with drink?

P: It makes me feel happy, confident, and I fit in with my friends.

HW: Ok, three things. Anything bad from drinking?

P: Yes, quarrels with my wife, trouble at work, and it is expensive.

HW: Does it have any negative or positive effects on your mood?

P: Yes, it makes me feel good at first but then I feel bad.

HW: OK, so that is three good things and four bad things.

P: OK, I can see that.

HW: What do you think of that?

P: OK, I can see that maybe I hadn't looked at the bad side of it but don't feel ready to change now.

HW: OK so maybe come back again another time or whenever you feel ready, and we can talk about how you might want to stop or reduce – any questions?

P: No, that is clear and thanks for not giving me a lecture about drinking being bad for me.

11 Mental State and Mini-Mental State Examination

Examining a mental state and practising it can assist a health worker to make appropriate professional assessments and referrals. Understanding how to examine and document appearance and behaviour, speech, mood, thoughts, delusions and hallucinations and how to describe them, as well as the concept of insight, are important parts of a mental health assessment. This can be a challenge in a primary care setting where time is usually limited. Clinics in some areas may have from 25 to over 100 people attending each day. However, with practice, assessing mental state can become quite quick with the development of good communication skills.

The Mini-Mental State Examination (MMSE, Folstein et al. 1975)[14] of cognitive state is also taught as the core assessment in suspected dementia.

12 Spiritual Beliefs and the Place of Prayer

Prayer and spiritual beliefs and rituals form a key role in the lives of many people around the world. Many people and communities get a lot of comfort from their spiritual beliefs and rituals. Asking about religious faith and practices in health care form part of holistic psychosocial care. The role of the volunteer is to acknowledge and respect people's religious and non-religious views, whatever their own personal beliefs, and to not impose their own views on others . The sense of community in religious life can also be a powerful support to many people, particularly during difficult times. Sometimes discussions can lead to concerns about evil spirits which may call for sensitivity and care and the assistance of local colleagues.

Table 9.12 Some additional useful considerations

How to manage hyperventilation and panic attacks
One technique, based on what underwater divers use, is to demand maintenance of eye contact with the patient. Starting with 'Look at me' and then mirroring the person's fast breathing is followed by slowly reducing the speed and depth of breathing, reassuring the person that they are doing well and have enough air. At the same time, ask them to feel their feet grounding them to the earth.
Alternatively, cupping hands around the mouth can be effective. Demonstrations help participants to understand how simply these techniques can be used and taught.

Attending to specific needs that work well for individuals
Volunteers have found that each person is actually their own source of expertise on their recovery. This is for patients as well as health workers. Exploring what works for each person can be rewarding. Asking how the person coped last time they had a crisis is usually revealing and therapeutic.

Addressing maladaptive strategies and healthy living
When patients and health workers develop their own coping strategies based on what works for them, they may make unhealthy choices, such as substance misuse or overworking. Addressing these individual habits and education about maladaptive coping is part of psychosocial intervention.

Other therapies and approaches
- Cognitive behavioural therapy[15]
- WHO manual Thinking Healthy[16]
- Group interpersonal therapy[17]
- Doing What Matters in Times of Stress[18]
- Problem Management Plus[19]

13 Overall Well-Being

Attention to exercise, nutrition, sleep, reproductive health and smoking is necessary as part of the overall psychosocial approach and support.

Other useful considerations are provided in Table 9.12.

Conclusion

Simple teaching approaches and interventions can have a significant impact on the quality of a consultation between a health worker and a patient and their family. The toolkit described uses a variety of techniques to help equip health workers with basic skills and provide cheap or free interventions which can be taught or provided to patients. The value of psychosocial interventions cannot be underestimated. This includes prescribing medication.

References

1 World Health Organization.mhGAP Intervention Guide, version 2. Geneva: WHO; (2016). www.who.int/mental_health/publications/mhGAP_intervention_guide/en/#:~:text=The%20mhGAP%20Intervention%20Guide%20%28mhGAP-IG%29%20for%20mental%2C%20neurological,by%20WHO%20to%20assist%20in%20implementation%20of%20mhGAP.

2 Volunteering and International Psychiatry Special Interest Group (VIPSIG). www.rcpsych.ac.uk/members/special-interest-groups/volunteering-and-international (accessed 30.12.2020).

3 World Health Organization and UNHCR. mhGAP Humanitarian Intervention Guide. Geneva: WHO; (2015). www.who.int/mental_health/publications/mhgap_hig/en/.

4   Patel V & Hanlon C. Where There Is No Psychiatrist: A Mental Health Care Manual (2nd ed.). Cambridge: Royal College of Psychiatrists; 2018.

5   World Health Organization. Problem Management Plus (PM+). Geneva: WHO; (2016). http://apps.who.int/iris/bitstream/1 0665/206417/1/WHO_MSD_MER_16.2_e ng.pdf?ua=1.

6   Caldwell PHY, Nankivell G, Sureshkymar P. Simple behavioural interventions for nocturnal enuresis in children. Cochrane Database of Systematic Reviews. (2013). DOI:10.1002/14651858. CD003637.pub3.

7   WHO, War and Trauma Foundation and World Vision International. Psychological First Aid: A Guide for Field Workers. Geneva: WHO; (2011). http://whqlibdoc .who.int/publications/2011/9789241548205 _eng.pdf?ua=1.

8   International Medical Corps Training Videos. www.youtube.com/channel/UCxqgY l55Bt3s7a_BATcLw7w (accessed 30.12.2020).

9   Davis DM & Hayes JA. What are the benefits of mindfulness? A practice review of psychotherapy-related research. Psychotherapy. 2011; 48(2), 198–208. http s://doi.org/10.1037/a0022062.

10 Harsora P, Kessmann J. Nonpharmacologic management of chronic insomnia. American Family Physician. 2009 Jan 15;79 (2),125–30. PMID: 19178064.

11 World Health Organization. ASSIST. The Alcohol, Smoking and Substance Involvement Screening Test. Geneva: WHO; (2010). https://apps.who.int/iris/bit stream/handle/10665/44320/978924159938 2_eng.pdf;jsessionid=9EA3DBFA0343A41

D50382E363AC7D72B?sequence=1 (accessed 29.10.2020).

12 Prochaska JO & DiClemente CC. Stages and processes of self-change of smoking, toward an integrative model of change. Journal of Consulting and Clinical Psychology. 1983;51,390–95. doi:10.1037/0022-006X.51.3.390.

13 Miller WR & Rollnick S. Applications of Motivational Interviewing. Motivational Interviewing: Helping People Change (3rd ed.). Guilford Press; 2013.

14 Folstein Marshal F, Folstein Susan E, McHugh Paul R. 'Mini-mental state': a practical method for grading the cognitive state of patients for the clinician, Journal of Psychiatric Research. 1975; 12;189–98, https://doi.org/10.1016/0022-3956(75) 90026-6.

15 Sheldon B. Cognitive-Behavioural Therapy: Research and Practice in Health and Social Care. Routledge; 2011.

16 World Health Organization. Thinking healthy: a manual for psychosocial management of perinatal depression, WHO generic field-trial version 1.0. World Health Organization; 2015.

17 World Health Organization. Group interpersonal therapy (IPT) for depression. World Health Organization; 2016.

18 World Health Organization. Doing what matters in times of stress: an illustrated guide; 2020.

19 World Health Organization. Problem Management Plus (PM+): individual psychological help for adults impaired by distress in communities exposed to adversity. World Health Organization; 2016.

Further Useful Reading

Casañas R, Catalán R, Penadés R et al. Evaluation of the effectiveness of a psychoeducational intervention in treatment-naïve patients with antidepressant medication in primary care: a randomised controlled trial. Scientific World Journal 2015. https://doi.org/10.1155/2015/ 718607.

Engel GL. The need for a new medical model: a challenge for biomedicine. Science 1977;196:129–36.

Griffiths KM, Carron-Arthur B, Parsons A et al. Effectiveness of programs for reducing the stigma associated with mental disorders. A meta-analysis of randomised controlled trials. World Psychiatry 2014 Jun;13(2): 161–75. doi: 10.1002/wps.20129. PMID: 24890069; PMCID: PMC4102289.

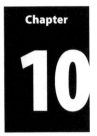

After the Trip: Coming Home and Sustainability

Peter Hughes

Introduction

This chapter considers the transition back to UK life, supervision possibilities and the sustainability of any project after the volunteer returns home. Sustainability needs to be worked through at all stages of any project but often comes to the fore in the 'after' phase. There is usually a lot of focus on getting people prepared for their volunteering and what to do whilst they are away from the UK. However, the 'after the trip' phase can be particularly difficult for some. At a minimum, there is a kind of reverse culture shock to be back in the UK.

To aid an understanding of this return period, a survey was conducted along with interviews with a sample of volunteers at the Royal College of Psychiatrists. The volunteers were asked to recall and reflect on their adjustments upon return. Using this, the chapter discusses some specific examples, which bring together common themes, and summaries are provided below.

What Does Coming Home Mean?

What happens after you have been away volunteering for a few weeks or a few months, or even some years? There are psychological, work, home, family and practical adjustments to be made.

For some people, they have got 'the bug' and have a growing desire to undertake further global voluntary placements. Some make a career decision to work in global health. Others try to work in the two worlds of global mental health and the NHS. There are some, just a few, who had the experience and never want to repeat it. However, there is rarely any regret at having had the experience.

For many volunteers, the experience is transformative, it will stay with them for the rest of their lives and is remembered as one of the highlights of their careers. Volunteers reflecting on their experiences often speak of the people they worked with, the patients they met, their impact on the lives of people they worked with and their hopes for sustainability. Fortunately, people forget about the heat, the bugs and the lack of home comforts or recall them with amusement and good humour.

Psychological Adjustment

Personally, a common theme in those after the trip is a psychological readjustment to being back in the UK. Psychological responses are common, with mixed emotions on return[1]. There is a reverse culture shock. There is the relief of being back home. However, the volunteer may feel like they are living in two different worlds for quite a while.

Life may seem boring at times. The volunteer may feel under-utilised compared to their tasks overseas.

This can be a very isolating experience as the volunteer has half their mind in the UK and half back where they were. Others around them in the UK cannot really share this experience as it is unique. A health worker can be in an emergency setting or refugee camp one day and back in the UK on another. It is hard to leave that experience behind and others often cannot understand it without having been through that themselves. One volunteer stated, 'no one can understand what it was like and yet we have to carry on with our usual job with two worlds going on in our heads and wishing that we were helping back there'. A debrief is important on return to the UK. This can help transition back to usual life. This can be done by their UK-based supervisor ideally. The debriefing after return often focuses on technical issues but should encompass all areas the volunteer wants to talk through. It is important for the volunteer to understand that these reactions are very normal.

Symptoms of depression and anxiety are common transitory reactions on return to the UK after an initial euphoria phase. Volunteers may need to be aware of the impact of such symptoms. For example, there may be some strain on relationships. These are short-term changes and people return to normal functioning pretty quickly. There is no easy solution to this. Stress management may be helpful but just understanding that this is a short-term reaction is useful.

These challenges can be complicated by practical issues such as finding new accommodation, debts, conflict with others and guilt about having taken time off.

Some of the respondents to the Royal College of Psychiatrists survey and interviewees found it easier to adjust when they were able to still connect with their host countries with ongoing online projects, for example. This is a reflection of the development of a relationship with their hosts and the desire to continue to maintain this and to further contribute. It is through these maintained relationships that sustainable development can happen.

For many volunteers going to other countries, there is a need to change pace from a 'top gear' in the NHS to a slower gear. Many volunteers initially find the pace in the host countries frustrating. One of the areas of learning from global volunteering is to slow down for one's own health, well-being and for patient care back in the UK.

Volunteers need to work on making use of the experience for their own professional development back in the NHS. This is an individual path in using skills of leadership, transcultural psychiatry, resource management, and to be ambassadors of global volunteering.

Generally there are less effects on return to work, as it can distract from psychological processes. For some, there may be frustration at the disparity between resources in the UK and low- and middle-income countries (LMICs). The stark juxtaposition of resources in the UK NHS against what was present in a low-income country can take a while to overcome. Others may feel exhausted and value a holiday before resuming work.

At home, there may be tensions as volunteers settle back home. They may feel the urge to travel again which can be a cause of tension with family. Couples may need to reboot their relationship. Couples who volunteer together may find it easier to settle back to UK life.

Volunteers' experiences – case examples

These stories are representative of just some of the many experiences and capture some common themes. The longer the person is away and the more complex the assignment, the longer the period of time that is needed to adjust back to life in the UK.

Case 1

This doctor describes volunteering in a number of countries including Somaliland and Malawi in a very well-structured programme. What the volunteer was particularly happy with was being able to continue work online after returning to the UK and maintain relationships with new colleagues. This helped adjustment back to UK work. In particular, the volunteer learned about teaching skills, culture, barriers to recovery and about his own character. These were all areas the volunteer could put into practice in the UK. The volunteer was very happy to be able to talk of experiences and share these with others in the UK. It was hard at times to explain to others really what it was like.

This was consolidated by other projects. Some were intensive and others less so. The volunteer found that doing so allowed a 'lived experience' of global work. However, coming back to the UK was like a crash landing and took some time to adjust. The volunteer found the NHS to be a comforting, familiar environment and over time was able to make use of his learned experiences. These projects were as a trainee and the volunteer recalled that many of the consultant interview questions subsequently asked were about experiences as a global volunteer. The volunteer was able to highlight leadership, flexibility and the ability to use other experiences back in the NHS.

Case 2

This volunteer described the missions undertaken in several humanitarian contexts as very rewarding but exhausting. The transition back to UK NHS work was challenging and exhausting. The first few weeks were very difficult, and the volunteer felt that he was not 'all there'. In retrospect, the volunteer wonders if he may not have been up to par. This was unexpected and, in retrospect, the volunteer wished that he had taken a holiday on return to help with adjustment. At times, the volunteer wanted to talk about the experiences but did not feel others were interested, except superficially. It helped the volunteer to share with people who had had similar experiences. The volunteer now recognises with the passage of time the self-growth achieved clinically, in confidence, teaching skills, leadership and feeling inspired. On reflection, the volunteer recommends avoiding on-calls soon after returning to the UK. There was also a realisation about how worried his family were and, being somewhat older now, he may not take the same risks again.

Case 3

In another case, the volunteer had been away for a longer period of time. They needed to organise their accommodation back in the UK and deal with their finances. They felt a bit low in mood for a while. Although this volunteer had been able to develop many leadership skills, the volunteer felt somewhat deskilled clinically on return to the UK. Suddenly they were a small fish in a big pond, having been a big fish when they were away. Their family put some pressure on them not to go away again. However, the volunteer did wish to volunteer again in the future for further projects.

Table 10.1

After the trip tips

- Every reaction is different
- Have a debrief with someone who has had global health experience
- You may feel transitory symptoms of anxiety, depression and culture shock
- Use any opportunity to talk about your experiences formally and informally
- Try to continue relationships with host country and continue the work online
- Write a report that you can come back to with recommendations
- Connect with others with similar experiences online and face to face
- Some need a holiday soon after return to refresh themselves
- Establish routine and structure
- Set new goals and objectives
- Don't expect others to ask about your experiences
- Reflect on a job well done and now a new start

Practical

Practical issues are discussed in Chapters 8 and 9. Some volunteers may need to find accommodation on return, deal with debts or get new jobs. This needs to be planned for even before volunteering overseas. One common issue is interviews coming up when the volunteer is overseas. Skype interviews may be possible. There is no doubt that this return may raise many practical issues but with good planning these problems can be minimised.

Supervision

It is clear that the global volunteer requires supervision when they are engaged in a project. In addition, there are many volunteering projects that involve that same volunteer supervising others. Here we are referring to the volunteer providing supervision of health workers even after the volunteer has returned to their home in the UK. Supervision of health workers in their home countries by volunteers is one of the increasing areas of volunteering and will probably increase with the growth of online-based work.

Supervision is an essential part of the sustainability of many global mental health projects. It is one of the reasons for the failure of many projects. Supervision needs to be built into many projects from the beginning. It needs to be planned and included in the budget. Every volunteer needs to check that there is a supervision plan in place to make sure that it is a sustainable project. There is a need to think about how your presence can be meaningful in the longer term. Supervision is for everyone's benefit – the volunteers as well as the health workers and their patients.

Supervision structures may take time to build locally and hence continuing with support from the UK may be helpful to encourage the confidence of key interested people to take forward developments in services. For volunteers, one of the main interventions is training, and supervision is an essential component when the classroom work has finished. This needs a clear plan with a timetable of who will supervise whom, when and for how long.

Supervision and ongoing support can be provided by online platforms, webinars or return visits[2]. Of course, the ideal is local supervision by local health workers. It is unquestionable that face-to-face supervision is best. With limited resources it can be done by phone, internet or as peer supervision. An example of peer supervision is that of the psychiatric nurses in Sierra Leone[3]. Several times a year they were assembled together and facilitated supervision sessions enabling learning from each other. This was helpful for information and skill-sharing, and also to ensure skills of IT and data collection. UK volunteers can more easily supervise from a distance when connection is available online.

There are challenges to setting up and continuing supervision from the UK, not least of which are reliable internet connection, time differences and suitable time set aside by busy clinicians who may be unfamiliar with the concept of supervision and need reassurance and good experiences to value such support. Field experiences in the following chapters illustrate efforts made to offer supervision and the difficulties in making substantial continuing connections, for example the Sudan distance project. This programme of distance supervision followed face-to-face training. This was a volunteer project where UK psychiatrists supervised family doctors in Sudan, and it was perceived as useful when formally evaluated[4].

What tends to happen currently with supervision programmes is a high dropout rate but is rated as helpful for those that persevere. College volunteers have been involved in supervision online projects in countries including Ukraine, Bangladesh and Turkmenistan.

Clinical accountability is overcome by referring to standard national guidelines and ensuring that the health worker works things out for themselves, guided by manuals or other materials and not expecting direct clinical advice from the UK.

It is clearly so much better for appropriate clinical care for local practitioners to be receiving supervision first from local colleagues, which also helps support appropriate referral pathways and advice about ongoing clinical care suitable for the systems arrangements in each country. Distance supervision can complement this. Hence, perhaps our most useful work might be in training the trainers and assisting them in setting up sustainable pathways of supervision in their area.

Mentoring

Mentoring is very much related to supervision. This may cover more professional development areas and even personal areas, if appropriate. Many UK psychiatrists have a mentoring relationship with international colleagues and health workers with whom they have developed relationships over several years. Often these are mutually beneficial and supportive partnerships. There have been some online pairings with varying degrees of success. There are also opportunities for research and academic development. There is a rich opportunity for global online mentoring in the future and ideally this could lessen the 'brain drain' for low-income countries.

Sustainability

Sustainability is one of the principles of good global mental health work. There is a need to think about how your presence can be meaningful in the longer term. Many would argue that it takes several years to make sustainable changes. It really needs to be thought through how any project can have a real long-term effect. Sustainability is established in the preparation phase and every activity during a project should have sustainability in mind; at the least it is investment in human resources and capacity building.

Ways to support sustainability include:

—Following Government Policies

Sustainability can be driven by government policy and plans. Local champions may drive them forward through their interest. Following national principles and priorities will give a drive to sustainability.

—Financial Resourcing

Financial resources are one of the main ways of keeping a project going. There are times when projects can be linked for mutual benefit. For example, mental health may be linked to non-communicable diseases (NCDs). People with mental illness have an increased rate of NCDs and die earlier than other people. In this way, a project on one of the NCDs, such as diabetes or asthma, may have an embedded mental health component.

In some of the examples in this book we had projects that we had hoped the government would wish to continue as part of their plans. Sometimes that happens but, unfortunately, when the money runs out, often the project often comes to an end.

—Links with Universities and Institutions

This can be a way of ensuring sustainability through embedding programmes academically. Long-term links to UK academics and ongoing volunteer relationships is another way. Sustainability is helped by long-term institutional links. In this book we describe examples of Somaliland[5] and Malawi[6] where there have been long standing institutional links to UK. Other examples are mhGAP programmes which are part of the national priorities of many countries which drive sustainability[7]. The mental health plan may include mhGAP and have indicators around this. Advice on health systems, leadership, research skills, health records, pharmacy procurement and human rights issues, such as ensuring confidentiality of clinics, can be usefully offered.

—Training Individuals

Health workers trained in mental health benefit from the training offered. As is normal with any training (particularly one-offs), some parts of the content may become distant memories in time. The aim is to transfer some key and important content and principles. Reminder messages, top-up revision and supervision can really cement sustainable change.

Interventions may not only be in clinical areas but could also be in support with clinical records, health system strengthening, IT and human resources. Here systems can be changed that can increase sustainability. However, there are so many examples one can give where sustainable change happened at individual levels.

Health workers have shared their experiences of how they have learned something new that they can use to improve their patient care such as principles of treatment or even confidentiality. During training, one can see sometimes that some people really 'get it' and patients will be better off. They will start working in a different way. They may also teach others about a training model.

—Local Champions and Fostering Local Groups

A way of ensuring sustainability is fostering local champions of certain areas; for example, supporting a lead in rational prescribing to avoid polypharmacy. Unfortunately, champions of mental health can leave or move on, so it may be worth helping to build a local supportive group of professionals who can rely on each other for personal support and supervision. With increasing electronic capacity, colleagues in very different geographic locations can be helped to create a space for collaboration, listening, learning and sharing. This support can continue after volunteers are no longer involved. Building a group that supports integration of important cultural practices within new ways of working may be useful. Coupled with individual and group/peer support and supervision this can be a way of ensuring sustainable change.

–Maintaining Professional Standards

Using evidence-based, easily accessible culturally appropriate material, working with sustainable development goals, writing accurate reports and contributing to publications, building and maintaining collegiate relationships with host partners, are all within the remit of volunteers and necessary aid to sustainability.

Table 10.2 contains some tips for sustainability but is not a complete list.

Conclusion

Global mental health volunteering can be transformative, but we often do not adequately support the 'after the trip' phase. This is crucial to help people get back into social and professional NHS work. In doing so, they may be better placed to maximise their ability to use their newly learned skills. Key aspects to consider and mitigate include the psychological and work-based challenges upon return. Supervision, mentorship and debriefing can help with some of these transitions. Attention to the sustainability of volunteer work remains a key element for every phase of global mental health.

Table 10.2 Tips on sustainability

- Start thinking about this from the preparation phase
- Invest in people and invest in local and national champions
- Use evidence-based easily accessible culturally appropriate training materials
- Encourage volunteers to continue project involvement through online systems after they leave
- Submit report at end of assignment with details of how sustainable change has been effected and how hosts can continue to embed this
- Build project along with national mental health priorities so it may continue with local government support
- Partner with local NGOs and government
- Develop long-term relationship/partnership between UK institution and host country institutions – to allow return visits and online support
- Build SDGs and World Mental Health Action plan into projects
- Consider fundraising in the UK to support the project continuing and sustaining
- Bring and donate books and build online resources
- Build into academic programmes, for example a master's degree
- Consider publications of work to ensure there can be a drive to continue it (co-authored and developed)
- Remember the ethos of the partnership
- Support the development of research, audit and publications by international colleagues

References

1. Hughes P. UK mental health professionals volunteering in LMIC – benefits to UK and host countries; 2015.

2. Aboaja A, Myles P, Hughes P. Mental health e-supervision for primary care doctors in Sudan using the WHO mhGAP Intervention Guide. BJPsych International. 2015;12(S1):S-16-S-9.

3. Harris D, Wurie A, Baingana F et al. Mental health nurses and disaster response in Sierra Leone. The Lancet Global Health. 2018;6(2): e146-e7.

4. Ali S, Saeed K, Hughes P. Evaluation of a mental health training project in the republic of the Sudan using the mental health gap action programme curriculum. International Psychiatry. 2012;9(2):43–5.

5. King's Health Partners. King's Somaliland Partnership. www.kingshealthpartners.org/resources/case-studies/21-kings-somaliland-partnership.

6. Scotland-Malawi Mental Health Education Project. Malawi quick guide to mental health. SMMHEP.

7. World Health Organization. mhGAP intervention guide for mental, neurological and substance use disorders in non-specialized health settings: mental health Gap Action Programme (mhGAP). version 2.0 ed. Geneva: World Health Organization; 2016.

Other Resources and References of Interest

Rose N, Hughes P, Sherese Ali et al. Integrating mental health into primary health care settings after an emergency: lessons from Haiti. Intervention 2011, Volume 9, Number 3, p. 211.

Patel V, Minas H, Cohen A et al. Global Mental Health. Oxford University Press; 2014.

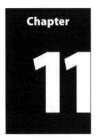

Monitoring, Evaluation and Research

Sam Gnanapragasam and Dinesh Bhugra

Overview

Monitoring, evaluation and research offer ways to collect, analyse and learn from information to ensure effectiveness and guide improvement for future practice. This chapter outlines the importance of monitoring, evaluation and research when undertaking voluntary projects, and it considers best practice. It also considers the different aspects of a voluntary placement that a prospective volunteer should consider evaluating.

Ethical considerations should be explicitly considered when seeking to undertake monitoring, evaluation and research as part of volunteering. The first purpose of global volunteering is to offer support. Research should only be done with local partners in their interests as, otherwise, there is a risk that volunteering results in extractive research practice done for the sole benefit of the global volunteer/researcher will have limited benefits for host individuals, partner organisations and communities.

Often, monitoring, evaluation and research are thought of as the same thing. Whilst there is overlap, each has a specific meaning and purpose.

- Monitoring: collection of data that measures progress toward achieving programme objectives. It is used to track changes in programme performance over time[1].
- Evaluation: how well the programme activities have met expected objectives and/or the extent to which changes in outcomes can be attributed to the programme or intervention[1].
- Research: intended to prove a theory or hypothesis and is more interested in producing generalisable knowledge[2].

Monitoring and evaluation (M&E) are often grouped together and have distinct characteristics to that of research. Table 11.1 outlines the differences between research and evaluation as demonstrated by Cohen and colleagues.

Monitoring and Evaluation (M&E)

M&E should take place throughout an assignment and feed into project sustainability. It is important to plan the M&E from the beginning. This must include both the M&E of the voluntary roles themselves as well as the project impact (see section on scope below). There are specific tools available such as the IASC Common Monitoring and Evaluation Framework for Mental Health and Psychosocial Support in Emergency Settings (version 2.0)[4] but it is possible to create a tailored M&E tool oneself.

Ideally M&E considerations should be incorporated from the planning phase, as often the outcomes and metrics will help clarify the project aim/objectives. Starting early in this

Table 11.1 Differences and similarities of research and M&E, from Cohen and colleagues[3]

Features	Research	Monitoring and evaluation
Audiences	Disseminated widely and publicly	Often commissioned and becomes the property of the sponsors; not for the public domain
Data sources and types	More focused body of evidence	Has a wide field of coverage (e.g. costs, benefits, feasibility, justifiability, needs, value for money) – so tends to employ a wider and more eclectic range of evidence from an array of disciplines and sources than research
Decision-making	Used for macro decision-making	Used for micro decision-making
Focus	Concerned with how something works	Concerned with how well something works
Origins	From scholars working in a field	Issued from/by stakeholders
Outcome focus	May not prescribe or know its intended outcomes in advance	Concerned with the achievement of intended outcomes
Participants	Less (or no) focus on stakeholders	Focuses almost exclusively on stakeholders
Politics of the situation	Provides information for others to use	May be unable to stand outside the politics of the purposes and uses of (or participants in) an evaluation
Purposes	Contributes to knowledge in the field, regardless of its practical application; provides empirical information – i.e. 'what is' Conducted to gain, expand and extend knowledge; to generate theory, 'discover' and predict what will happen	Designed to use the information/ facts to judge the worth, merit, value, efficacy, impact and effectiveness of something – i.e. 'what is valuable' Conducted to assess performance and to provide feedback; to inform policy-making and 'uncover'. The concern is with what has happened or is happening
Relevance	Can have wide boundaries (e.g. to generalise to a wider community); can be prompted by interest rather than relevance	Relevance to the programme or what is being evaluated is a prime feature. Has to take particular account of timeliness and particularity
Reporting	May include stakeholders/ commissioners of research – but may also report more widely (e.g. in publications)	Reports to stakeholders and commissioners of research

Table 11.1 (cont.)

Features	Research	Monitoring and evaluation
Scope	Often (though not always) seeks to generalise (external validity) and may not include evaluation	Concerned with the particular – e.g. a focus only on specific programmes. Seeks to ensure internal validity and often has a more limited scope
Stance	Active and proactive	Reactive
Standards for judging quality	Judgments are made by peers, standards for which include validity, reliability, accuracy, causality, generalisability, rigour	Judgments are made by stakeholders, standards for which also include utility, feasibility, involvement of stakeholders, side effects, efficacy, fitness for purpose
Status	An end in itself	A means to an end
Time frames	Often ongoing and less time-bound: although this is not the case with funded research	Begins at the start of a project and finishes at its end
Use of results	Designed to demonstrate or prove. Provides the basis for drawing conclusions, and information on which others might or might not act – i.e. it does not prescribe Based in social science theory – i.e. is 'theory dependent'	Designed to improve. Provides the basis for decision-making; might be used to increase or withhold resources or to change practice
Use of theory	Creates the research findings	Not necessary to base in theory; is 'field dependent' – i.e. derived from the participants, the project and stakeholders May (or may not) use research findings

process will also ensure that the evaluation design will be most robust, and therefore the resultant data of higher quality and more useful in the longer term. If left too late and considered as an 'add-on' towards the end of the project or voluntary placement, then the evaluation and data gathered will have a number of constraints and limitations.

It is also important to note that where the project or your voluntary trip has been funded, particularly if it has been done so by large-scale global health funding organisations and related grants, there will often be stringent requirements to provide an evaluation plan as part of submission of the proposal and upon completion.

The process may be challenging and may feel at times like it is added work. It may also feel relatively unimportant work with other seemingly more important competing demands, for example delivery teaching or providing care. However, M&E is important for a number of reasons. It is necessary as part of an active cycle to ensure that there is:

a) Service development
b) Understanding of current and future resourcing (including funding) efficiency and requirements
c) Informed decisions about this and future programmes
d) A voice and view of stakeholders/participants/patients in the project implementation and future ways of working

Where possible, it is helpful to bring a positive outlook to the M&E process to ensure best outcomes and buy-in from colleagues as this will be beneficial to the project, all stakeholders and you.

Shared Language and Key Terms

As an international volunteer, you will be working with and alongside a range of national, international and voluntary organisations. Each will have their own M&E approaches and techniques. As such, it is helpful to have an understanding of terminology used and how it is understood in the IASC framework around MHPSS to ensure that you are using the same nomenclature[4].

When considering M&E, there is a subtle but important difference between what is considered as monitoring and evaluation. See Figure 11.1.

Key Definitions

Indicators specific items to be measured. They may be quantitative (e.g.number of users) or qualitative (e.g. experience of users).

Activities 'actual work' done and implemented.

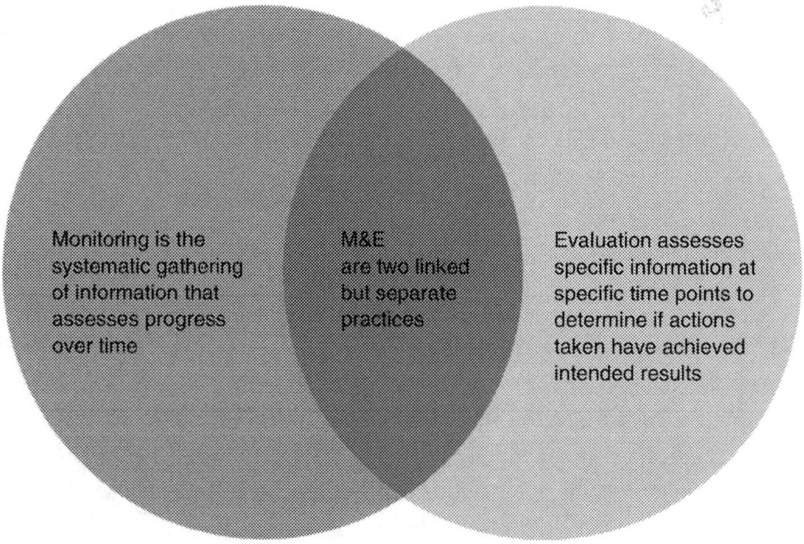

Monitoring is the systematic gathering of information that assesses progress over time

M&E are two linked but separate practices

Evaluation assesses specific information at specific time points to determine if actions taken have achieved intended results

Figure 11.1 Differences between monitoring and evaluation, from the NCVO Charities Evaluation Service[5].

Outcomes	the resultant impact of the activities undertaken, and the resultant changes.
Goal	the desired end result if the project delivers activities and the outcomes are met. For example, a goal might be to reduce mental health impact of conflict on internally displaced people in a particular region.

Scope and Areas to Evaluate

Project Evaluation

Project evaluations are methodical and are objective assessments of an ongoing or completed project. Specific aspects to consider when undertaking an evaluation include items such as:

o Completion of agreed goals and objectives
o Satisfaction of beneficiaries
o Satisfaction of host
o Efficiency related to resources used
o Patient impact – this can be difficult to measure and needs surveys and other techniques such as interviews or focus groups. Areas to consider include acceptability, functioning, well-being, mental health measures, social behaviour and social connectedness
o Sustainability plan in place and working

The host organisation and stakeholders need to provide some degree of leadership on this evaluation. Often however, this can be passed directly to you as the volunteer and UK sponsor/organisation. The project evaluation can be complemented by an end of project report.

Volunteer Evaluation

The volunteer, in terms of role, effectiveness and performance, is worth evaluating through-out the process. This can include the volunteer's own reflections and self-evaluation, as well as multi-source feedback from members of the team including supervisors, co-workers /volunteers and service recipients. Some organisations will have specific indicators. These may include:

o Reliability
o Diligence
o Trustworthiness
o Flexibility
o Administration and IT skills
o Achievement of goals
o Organisational skills

Participant Evaluation in Training Programmes

The volunteer should ensure that any training provided is evaluated, so as to ascertain impact and also ensure ongoing learning for future training delivery. Evaluations may wish to include:

o Pre- and post-test for assessment of knowledge at the beginning and end of training
o Further assessment of skills and practice through mock clinical scenarios
o Observation of participants performing tasks in groups or alone
o Evaluation of a training at the end through a feedback form

Clinical Evaluation and Related Capacity Building

This can be used for observing and training clinicians doing their usual work. It can mirror the workplace-based assessments of the Royal College of Psychiatrists. The volunteer can undertake an evaluation of the health worker in a clinic during on-the-job training and use this as a progress indicator. This is a useful tool for supervision.

The WHO and UNICEF have also recently developed 'EQUIP – Ensuring Quality in Psychological Support'[12]. This is a tool that has been designed to support those in the humanitarian and development settings to improve the consistency and quality of both training and service delivery. They have been tested across a range of countries including Ethiopia, Kenya, Lebanon, Peru and Nepal, with evidence that use of EQUIP resulted in training improvement.

Evaluation of longer-term effect on clinical practice and service development is a much harder task and really needs a comprehensive evaluation protocol to establish what has been effective and what made improvements possible.

Supervision

There are some tools that enable evaluation during supervision. Areas to consider in supervision include:

○ Capacity to engage with patients and show appropriate respect and care
○ Drug usage, administration and prescribing skills
○ Diagnostic coding
○ Psychosocial skills
○ Process metrics such as the number of cases of mental health seen per week

Evaluation Model

There are several considerations when developing the evaluation model for the project and voluntary placement. These relate to identifying the focus, evaluation question, recognising evaluation constraints, deciding the type of evaluation metrics to utilise (process versus impact), and how best to disseminate/utilise the findings.

1. Consider focus of evaluation and develop an evaluation question

   a. Before undertaking an evaluation, it is important to firstly determine the purpose of the evaluation and the project. By ensuring that this is undertaken at the starting point, this may allow for streamlining of both the evaluation and project.

   b. Engage stakeholders throughout the process to ensure that the evaluation plan is co-developed. This is crucial as indeed the priorities of the local stakeholders may be different, and content/tools acceptable may be varied. For example, it may be the case that focus groups do not work well or that reading/writing compression levels are varied, making written feedback challenging.

2. Determine constraints on evaluation. There may be a number of constraints, and these may relate to:

   a. Time and budget – an evaluation strategy undertaken by a specialist M&E team will be different in terms of time and resourcing when compared to one that will be conducted by you or a small team.

b. Data availability – wider data related to health service usage and population level data may not be available. As such, you may not always be able to measure outcome metrics (e.g. decrease in number of patients waiting for mental health support) and may need to instead rely on process metrics (e.g. number of people who are trained in diagnosing depression using mhGAP). Data availability is also challenging in culturally sensitive topics that may be seen as taboo or where an individual/family is worried about confidentiality. This may be more complicated when using translators and other local stakeholders.

c. Political/other factors and constraints – if you are hosted by a particular organisation, country or group, there may be some restrictions or limitations on the scope of the project. Political consideration and sensitivity are necessary. For example, certain groups may find negative feedback from the evaluations challenging and thus may opt to only publish positive findings (selective publishing).

3. Process or impact evaluation – consider whether the project is best suited to process evaluation (e.g. number of people who are trained in diagnosing depression using the mhGAP) or impact evaluation (e.g. decrease in number of patients waiting for mental health support).

a. Process evaluation – this considers the steps in the implementation of a project and uses those steps in the logic model to consider how successful the project is[6]. An example of a logic model is presented in Figure 11.2. Part of this includes determination of baseline measures and identification of target indicators (what will be measured through the evaluation).

b. Impact evaluation – this considers the impact of the project or placement in subsequent improvement in outcomes for the target population(s).

Research and Project Ownership

As noted in the definitions section above, research is different from M&E. Given the remit of research in seeking to analyse a hypothesis and generate generalisable evidence, it is not a formal and necessary part of a voluntary project in the same way that M&E is. Nonetheless, some volunteers may wish to undertake a research project. Further and increasingly, research is seen as a key way in which to work in global mental health and contribute to the improvement in population health. If wishing to undertake research, there are several key principles to consider. The field of global mental health research is vast, and this section does not explore this in depth but rather outlines key principles if wishing to undertake research.

Firstly, regardless of whether you intend to monitor and evaluate the project, or generate new evidence through a research study, the project should be undertaken in consultation and co-production with a range of stakeholders including the local community/proposed beneficiary of the project. This is crucial for not only ensuring relevance of the project, and sustainability, but also to balance the ownership of growth and research opportunities.

Secondly, the ownership of the project should also be reflected in the authorship as noted by a consensus statement on publication of research from international partnerships[8]. This is important as studies undertaken in low- and middle-income countries (LMICs) have been found to be predominated by authors from high-income countries[9]. Indeed, a different analysis found that 30% of primary research undertaken in LMICs did not

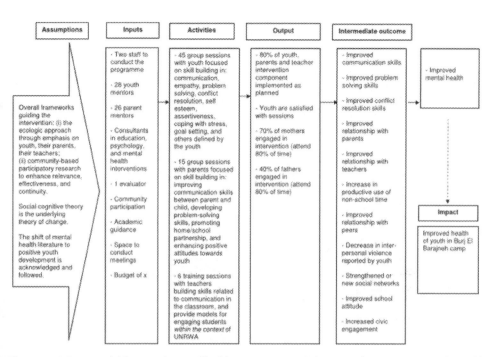

Figure 11.2 Logic model for a youth mental health intervention in a Palestinian refugee camp, Figure from Afifi and colleagues' study[7]

have a single local author[10]. Care should be taken against 'parachute' research whereby research is undertaken in LMICs without adequate recognition of local research, staff and supporting infrastructure[11].

Thirdly, in undertaking any research work, it is worth considering whether this could be used as an opportunity to further develop local research capacity and skills in the area. Such work could be done through formal teaching sessions or mentorship and lead to co-development of skills.

Fourthly, it is necessary to follow the best practice research standards in all settings – this includes the need to get ethical approval (local). At times, this may take a long time and, as such, considerable planning is needed prior to the research placement to ensure that this is possible. Again, such processes can be best navigated with the help and partnership of local expertise.

There are increasingly opportunities to undertake research, with the growth of global mental health as a discipline, centres of global mental health being established, master's courses on global mental health being available and with possibilities to undertake global health doctoral training/PhDs in this area. A notable example is the Wellcome funded CREATE PhD Programme that recruits five paired PhD fellows from the UK and host African countries each year.

Conclusions

Monitoring, evaluation and research should be considered and planned for from the outset when undertaking a global volunteering project or placement. The nature, scope and tools used to undertake this – particularly M&E, as this is necessary – should be co-developed with local partners. Such practices not only ensure that any work undertaken is evaluated for effectiveness, but also lessons can be learnt for the future, and principles of sustainability and accountability can be placed throughout the project and upon completion.

References

1. Global Health Learning Centre. Monitoring and evaluation (M&E). www.globalhealthlearning.org/taxonomy/term/1321.

2. Health Research Authority. Defining research table www.hra-decisiontools.org.uk/research/docs/DefiningResearchTable_Oct2017-1.pdf.

3. Cohen L, Manion L, Morrison K. Evaluation and Research. Research Methods in Education. Routledge; 2002. pp. 79–86.

4. IASC (Inter-Agency Standing Committee). The common monitoring and evaluation framework for mental health and psychosocial support in emergency settings: with means of verification (Version 2.0). Geneva: IASC; 2021.

5. The National Council for Voluntary Organisations. Charities evaluation services: about monitoring and evaluation. www.ncvo.org.uk/practical-support/consultancy/ncvo-charities-evaluation-services.

6. USAID (United States Agency for International Development). An evaluation framework for USAID-funded TIP prevention and victim protection programs; 2009.

7. Afifi RA, Makhoul J, El Hajj T et al. Developing a logic model for youth mental health: participatory research with a refugee community in Beirut. Health Policy and Planning. 2011;26(6):508–17.

8. Morton B, Vercueil A, Masekela R et al. Consensus statement on measures to promote equitable authorship in the publication of research from international partnerships. Anaesthesia. 2022;77(3):264–76.

9. Hedt-Gauthier BL, Jeufack HM, Neufeld NH et al. Stuck in the middle: a systematic review of authorship in collaborative health research in Africa, 2014–2016. BMJ Global Health. 2019;4(5):e001853.

10. Ghani M, Hurrell R, Verceles AC et al. Geographic, subject, and authorship trends among LMIC-based scientific publications in high-impact global health and general medicine journals: a 30-month bibliometric analysis. Journal of Epidemiology and Global Health. 2021;11(1):92.

11. The Lancet Global Health. Closing the door on parachutes and parasites. 2018. p. e593.

12. EQUIP: Ensuring Quality in Psychological Support. https://equipcompetency.org/en-gb.

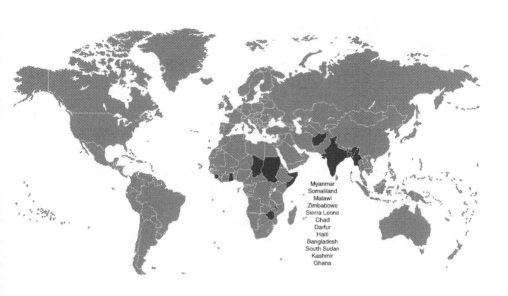

Myanmar
Somaliland
Malawi
Zimbabowe
Sierra Leone
Chad
Darfur
Haiti
Bangladesh
South Sudan
Kashmir
Ghana

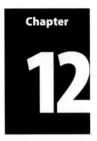

Myanmar: Mental Health Training, Recipient Perspective

Sai Kham Thaw

Introduction

This chapter solely reflects my experience and opinions on using the WHO mhGAP Intervention Guide[1] that I have participated in as a trainee as well as a volunteer facilitator.

I am a junior doctor working as a medical officer in Yangon, Myanmar. I met the Royal College of Psychiatrists (RCPsych) volunteer team at an mhGAP programme in Taunggyi in 2016 organised by the charity Mind to Mind Myanmar, Myanmar Medical Association GP Society and RCPsych. Later, I volunteered to help translate and co-facilitate the training from 2017 to 2019 in Mawlamyine, Pathein and Mandalay. This allowed me to work with trainers from the UK.

Experience as Trainee and Volunteer

Stigma for mental health is extensive in Myanmar. Patients and families are reluctant to seek help. They would rather turn to traditional medicine or regard the psychotic symptoms as spiritual problems or possessions and go to the monks, spiritual healers or mediums instead. Patients' family members are ashamed of them, and some try to hide them from the public eye. This results in a delay in seeking medical help and some patients' conditions have become serious by the time they reach general practitioners or psychiatrists. These patients are referred to two psychiatric hospitals (one in Yangon and another in Mandalay), 22 mental health wards of general hospitals or 35 mental health outpatient facilities[2,3]. There are extremely few specifically trained mental health nurses and social workers and less than 300 psychiatrists covering the whole country which has a population of 53.71 million. Hence, mental health training like the mhGAP programme is much needed for Myanmar as it is designed to help primary care practitioners manage mental ill-health in the community.

Doctors Training in Mental Health

Mental health training for doctors has been quite rare and educational opportunities were limited in Myanmar until recent years. In our medical undergraduate curriculum, psychiatry training was only for two weeks in the final clinical year. However, the new curriculum that started last year has more emphasis on psychiatry. Therefore, we as trainees did not know exactly how much we could expect from international trainers offering such programmes, but the experience exceeded our expectations. Previous experiences of volunteer healthcare educational programmes seemed superficial and insensitive to our cultural needs. However, since taking part in mhGAP lectures, small group discussions and role plays, we saw the time and effort that the volunteer trainers had put in for us and we acknowledged the mhGAP training as one of the best mental health workshops brought to Myanmar.

Importance of Language

Language is considered one of the top problems in this programme for the local trainees as English is not our mother tongue. Although the curriculum for the medical degree in Myanmar is in English, not all health professionals are fluent as written English is easier than speaking it. One of the things that the trainers did to help was to slow down the pace while speaking clearly and concisely. If the pace became too slow, this could sound condescending to the audience, but the trainers managed this well at the right tempo, in my opinion. It helped that a lot of the training was interactive. We had lectures as well as small group discussions and role plays. My role and that of other bilingual colleagues was to help interpret between the facilitators and the trainees. This helped to overcome the language barrier in large group lectures and small group discussions. I later joined the team not only to help translate but also to co-facilitate and take part in role plays.

Adaptation of Training to Clinical Practice

Some trainees thought the training would not be easy to adapt to their practice. The GP system in Myanmar is not organised like the NHS in the UK. Clinics are run independently by the doctors themselves, but they are not linked to local tertiary centres and are not government-funded. Patients are not registered with a single GP as in the UK and they have the option to go to government-run hospitals free of charge or see a private specialist. They can choose any clinic and pay the doctor directly. A problem in small cities is that patients refuse to pay for consultations unless they are given medication. As with many mental health issues, medication is not always necessary, and counselling and psycho-education may play a bigger role. Therefore, some trainees think that psychosocial interventions would not be helpful to them as their patients would not be willing to pay them. In my opinion, this will change over time as patients begin to experience the effectiveness of counselling and psycho-education.

Suicide and sexual assault cases are dealt with directly by the police in Myanmar. GPs are unable to help unless the victims are physically hurt and need immediate attention. Such patients are referred to government hospitals where it is hard to provide an environment with privacy. This is where they are interviewed by the police. Thus, the mental trauma is not supported well. Psychological first aid taught in the course introduced a different attitude to the approach of these cases and what we could do for victims as healthcare professionals while keeping in mind not to worsen the trauma they have suffered. This was delivered in the course as a role play and it portrayed effectively how we could apply it in a real-life situation. Although it just involved a simple act of kindness and providing basic needs, I felt that this was one of the most important aspects of the training.

Learning from the Experience

What I learnt from the programme helped a lot during my practice as a medical officer, especially with panic attacks and anxiety-related symptoms, medically unexplained symptoms, self-harm and depression. I find the 'hand technique' of psychosocial support (see

Chapter 9 Psychological Techniques) very useful and simple to teach to the patients regardless of their background and education. It allows me to encourage them to seek help from family and friends and know that they are not alone. Panic attacks and anxiety-related problems are the most frequent cases that I see in A&E. The training changed my approach by first taking time for the patient to calm down while providing a safe and private environment, rather than just prescribing lorazepam. Patients with medically unexplained symptoms with extensive investigation results are not uncommon in my everyday practice. In mhGAP training, I learnt how to really listen to the patients and help resolve their concerns. For instance, one lady was admitted with breathlessness and had multiple investigations done recently which were all normal. She was sure that there was something wrong with her and she switched from one specialist to another as she was told that everything was normal. She was taking more than eight vitamin supplements, was getting restless day by day as the cause was not found and was worried that she had cancer or some other disease. We discussed and explored all her concerns for about an hour. In our conversation, I recalled one thing from the training which was to understand and accept that patients can feel and suffer from symptoms even without a physical cause and that the troubled mind can also cause these symptoms. It was rewarding when she told me that I truly understood her.

Other trainees in the programme have told me that this training improved their clinical practice as they began to use the methods taught such as the 'hand technique', motivational interviewing and used star charts for behavioural problems. They shared how they enjoyed the role plays and found them exceedingly helpful as they were prompted on how to apply the techniques in their practice. One general practitioner trainee told us that more families came to consult with him after he practised family therapy role plays regarding children's problematic behaviour and the use of star charts to endorse good behaviour. He said that these families responded with good outcomes despite some of these parenting techniques being new to our culture. Another GP took more time talking to his patients, giving psycho-education and applied the skills acquired from the course. He said that this had helped him to connect with his patients as they opened up more, allowing him to make more accurate diagnoses, leading to better treatment outcomes.

Challenges

One of the challenges about the training course was the time frame as, personally, I felt that four days seemed a little short to cover the whole mhGAP handbook. It was hard to take in a lot of new information as well as a new attitude to mental health in such a short time and more practice would have been useful. However, the approach was to guide the trainees to use the book and was not about teaching the details. This only made sense to me after I assisted in the training as a volunteer. The participants came from different regions around the country. Unfortunately, the attendees missed out on valuable income by attending the course as they had to close their GP clinics. Hence, there was some reluctance to have longer training. The course was free, but GPs did have to cover travel and accommodation. Although this four-day time frame could not satisfy everyone, it remained the most reasonable amount of time to cover the course as well as to make it brief enough to meet the needs of the trainees.

Traditionally, it is our culture not to question teachers, who are held in high regard, so there was some reluctance to ask questions. The trainees always had queries regarding their practice, and these might even have been personal problems. However, they were more open towards the local trainers. Hence, it always helped to have at least one local trainer on the team. This assisted in relating the practice culturally. Some of the best training happened when local psychiatrists and their trainees attended, as this helped to forge local referral pathways.

It is best for the facilitator to try to avoid comparing religions and personal opinions about them. In one instance, one of the guest trainers talked in a small group discussion about how not to feel upset for the rest of the day if a very negative or aggressive patient comes to see you. However, he described it in a way that the negative 'vibe' comes from the patient and not from within us. This contradicted the Buddhist teachings which most influence our culture. The conversation led to a small argument, and it became a very awkward and uneasy situation. We managed to change the topic and move on with the training. It is not possible to know each and every opinion that might offend another's culture if we are not part of that community. However, it would be more effective to refrain from asserting strong opinions.

The biggest challenge may be the need for continued support and help from such programmes. Myanmar has been closed off from foreign help for about 50 years during the military regime. As much as we need help, especially in mental health, this help requires to be consistent. Volunteering work should not be a one-time thing. We need training like mhGAP to be continued over the years and those who complete the training may need refresher courses. Myanmar's mental health service is unbelievably limited in people power. We do not just need to educate the health personnel, but also need to raise awareness of mental health amongst the general public. Until recently in Myanmar, mental health services were mainly provided by general adult psychiatrists. Subspecialities such as forensic psychiatry, liaison psychiatry or neuropsychiatry are not yet well-organised. However, we are in the process of starting such developments. For instance, the first cohort of Child and Adolescent Mental Health Service-trained psychiatrists have already started working and the second cohort is finishing their training soon. In the future, we hope that there will be better development of different subspecialities and that the training can be adapted to better suit our culture.

We need every help to catch up with other countries and provide excellent care for our patients. Each mhGAP training may seem like just a little step but I can already see many changes in our practice, shifting towards a bigger difference.

References

1. World Health Organization. mhGAP Intervention Guide, www.who.int/publications/i/item/9789241549790.

2. Nguyen A, Lee C, Schojan M et al. Mental health interventions in Myanmar: a review of the academic and gray literature. Global Mental Health. 2018;5.

3. World Health Organization. Mental health atlas 2017. Geneva: World Health Organization; 2018. https://apps.who.int/iris/handle/10665/272735.

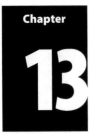

Myanmar: Mental Health Training, Trainer Perspective

Sophie Thomson

Visiting Myanmar

I first visited Myanmar in 1974 and managed to see this stunningly beautiful country even though internal travel was limited to a few ancient trains, some buses and run-down hotels. The floor of the YMCA and a church hall were offered as accommodation by kind but puzzled people, as only a handful of other Westerners visited Myanmar at that time.

Returning in 2015 was to another world, with modern hotels shooting up as tourist numbers multiplied, and international businesses had moved in. Yangon had become a patchwork of colonial buildings, new hotels and busy modern highways full of taxis. Buddhism remained a cornerstone of life for most people (Figure 13.1). The same old train to Mandalay, however, was still running on the same ancient tracks, while today's visitors are encouraged to fly on the many internal airlines instead of bouncing around all night on the sleeper train.

What remained noticeable was that people were still friendly, kind and willing to help, and we felt safer wandering around Yangon than in many other Asian cities. The younger demographic of Asia was immediately obvious, and the energy of a country moving at mind-boggling speed into the twenty-first century was palpable. It was exciting to be back and to have the opportunity to try make a contribution to the development of services for people with mental illness.

Training in mental health for GPs in primary care was set up and going well. In 2017, however, news about the violent atrocities in Rakhine State and the plight of the Rohingya people broke into international awareness and raised ethical concerns about the future of working in Myanmar. After much discussion and advice, the decision was made to continue working there, in a carefully planned way, for the well-being of people with mental illness.

The UK training team's personal experiences of travelling in Myanmar were that courtesy and respect abounded, and we felt comfortable and well cared for. We focused our energies on trying to make a contribution to capacity building of skills for professionals working in mental health and raising awareness of mental illness whenever we could. Residing in a living active Buddhist culture where kindness, courtesy and respect are practised was a real privilege. Watching young professionals understand mental health better and acquire skills was a delight.

The Myanmar Project

The Myanmar project started and was sustained by a Burmese graduate psychiatrist now living and working in UK. Bilingual and bicultural, she built a team of UK volunteers who prepared a programme and worked with hosts in Myanmar, organising the logistics of the training and working with partners in aligning expectations and sorting practicalities.

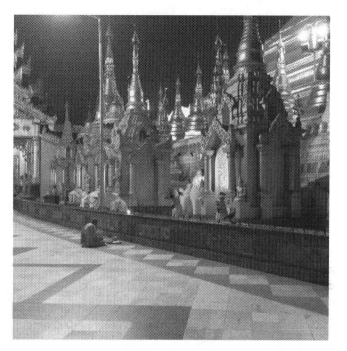

Figure 13.1 Shewdagon Pagoda Yangon

It took almost 18 months from our first meeting at a weekend mhGAP[1] orientation training in Manchester in the UK and getting excited about what might be possible, to arriving in Yangon to start training.

With an initial programme based primarily on the WHO mhGAP, the team included six volunteer psychiatrists from different specialties and a volunteer psychologist. Together we prepared pre- and post-training evaluations, as well as a further evaluation of changes in clinical practice one year later.

Training General Practitioners Based on WHO mhGAP

The Vice President of the Myanmar General Practitioner Society was keen to help general practitioners (GPs) access appropriate continuing professional development (CPD), and he agreed that training in the use of mhGAP would be most suitable. This guide is designed to enhance the skills of primary care practitioners in their interventions for mental, neurological and substance misuse disorders in non-specialised settings. We understood that precious little CPD was available for GPs in Myanmar, and medical student experience of mental illness had been limited to a few lectures in their final year. In terms of practice, they spent two weeks at overcrowded, large, old-style traditional psychiatric hospitals many miles outside the medical schools in central Yangon and Mandalay.

The participants were mainly young GPs eager to learn and they participated enthusiastically in interactive exercises, especially role plays, and seemed to enjoy the small group work where there were opportunities to speak in their own language. The four UK volunteers who did not speak Burmese worked with local psychiatry trainees who were kindly released from their usual duties by the senior psychiatrists.

Our hosts were always very polite and courteous and there were always food and drinks aplenty at every meeting and training event. Respect for older persons and especially teachers was obvious, and much appreciated!

Facebook is very popular in Myanmar, and word spread fast that this training was useful and enjoyable and free of charge. Requests for further training around the country resulted in plans for trainings in five more cities. After 5 years and 7 more visits of the UK team to Myanmar, a total of 11 mhGAP-based training programmes were successfully delivered.

Over 500 Burmese GPs have now had training in managing mental health in primary care. New friendships and informal support networks have been established for many GPs working single-handedly. Some GPs kindly participated in successive training programmes, helping also with language and cultural adaptation. Several Burmese psychiatry trainees also returned to join training teams on a regular basis. Working as co-trainers, they acquired skills to deliver the training themselves. Hopefully we have been part of training local champions of mental health who can contribute to developing services.

Evaluation, based on qualitative and quantitative measures of changes in clinical practice amongst the GPs at 3, 6 and 12 months after the end of their respective trainings, showed statistically significant improvements in their knowledge of mental health and their confidence in correct diagnosis and appropriate management. The toolkit of simple psychological skills, which had been developed for this project, was reported as particularly helpful. This research work is being prepared for publication.

Mental Health Care in Myanmar

Mental health care in Myanmar is based in large hospitals outside Yangon and Mandalay, with outpatients travelling there to follow-up clinics where appointments are often brief reviews of discharged patients. In other towns, outpatient services are now developing. Prescribed drugs need to be purchased and, although cheaper than in the UK, this can prove a burden for families. The situation has improved in recent years, but the possible poor compliance with long-term medication is concerning. Various local charities help out with the cost of drugs, and the environment is welcoming, with both hospitals laid out as separate buildings with gardens. The staff are caring and courteous, fostering an atmosphere of calm and kindness.

Most people with mental ill health receive little care in the community although GPs reported high rates of anxiety, stress and unexpected suicide. After training, GPs also reported an increased awareness of depression, usually presenting as somatic symptoms. They were bothered initially by the idea of talking about suicide but after practice they could see that this might actually help patients.

Stigma and shame about mental ill health, as in so many places and cultures around the world, pervades the community in Myanmar. Beliefs that evil spirits cause mental illness were reported as prevalent. One of our post-training evaluations showed that GPs reported that over 70% people with mental illness experienced stigma at some time and we heard how doctors interested in psychiatry also received stigmatising remarks.

The GPs also highlighted the time constraints of only a few minutes available per consultation. Moreover, patients usually expected the doctor to know best and to give them something that brought immediate relief. An emphasis on medication and the practice of administering vitamins, particularly by injection, was reported as widespread. They also commented that the culture discourages discussion of family problems and that ensuring privacy for consultations was often difficult.

At this stage, the project was being driven 'from the bottom up'. It was time to engage more active senior support, both professionally and organisationally. Helped by networks that our Burmese UK-based psychiatrists had built up over the years, the team met with senior academics and clinicians. This resulted in invitations in Yangon and Mandalay to introduce specialty training to psychiatrists.

Introduction to Subspecialties for Psychiatrists

There are currently fewer than 300 psychiatrists in Myanmar to serve a population of 53.7 million[2]. Therefore, considerable thought within the team and with our hosts was needed to decide how best to use the very limited days allocated to us. Senior psychiatrists and trainees were keen to hear about what happened in the UK and how services were developed. But would it be helpful to just tell them what we do in our context? What would be useful and interesting? What was realistic, given the current paucity of systematic community care, different social expectations and significantly limited resources in an already busy service?

As this was just the first step in a long road to development of services, we agreed that our aim should be to start a dialogue about mental health in the UK and Myanmar with an ethos of learning from each other. The participants spoke of their concerns about the current services for patients, especially those with substance misuse problems, and outlined their worries surrounding a legal requirement on doctors to report suicide attempts to the police. Moreover, they wanted to know how UK services manage the risk of harm when someone has a mental illness. Interestingly, they did not focus on child and adolescent mental health, despite an awareness of the accumulating stresses on young people growing up in a world very different to their parents. We wondered if this might be a reflection of the fact that the hospitals where they worked did not see children with mental health problems. Instead, this work fell to paediatricians.

The psychiatrists had ambitions for the future of mental health in Myanmar and were eager to hear about developments in the West. Some had idealised notions of mental health services in the UK. Their exposure to Western ways of managing many problems was largely based on reading articles and books about successful programmes and treatments. It was reassuring for them to hear from us about how much we often struggle to provide suitable care for many people with what often feels like inadequate resources.

We introduced some of the ways in which training in specialties are structured in the UK and together we discussed how these would need adaptation in Myanmar. In turn, the UK team was impressed by descriptions of how much work can be done by nurses and other skilled workers. While doctors in the UK can spend hours chasing up reports, filling out forms and endlessly hanging on the phone, our colleagues in Myanmar may well be using their time more appropriately.

Once again, it was essential to have Myanmar partners from the UK and locally, to help us engage in useful and culturally appropriate discussions. In a subsequent workshop, a generous UK trainer in research methods kindly gave an inspirational two-day workshop about the value and processes of research. His ability to teach and encourage was met with nods and excitement and ideas about possible publications. While psychiatrists in Myanmar may need support and help for this, the motivation certainly exists to move on with further academic pursuits. Hopefully we were not simply raising unrealistic expectations and that time, funds and support can be found to help these future leaders of mental health services participate in the development of services and join the world stage of global mental health.

As with the GPs, we found that the Myanmar psychiatrists were concerned about possible shortfalls in their training and clinical skills. Many were particularly keen to learn about psychological treatments and how to start using them with their patients. After much consultation, we ran a three-day workshop in Mandalay as an introduction to psychotherapy, focusing on psychological techniques useful for short consultations. There were also practice sessions on inpatient group work, and an introduction to Cognitive Behavioural Therapy (CBT). These beginnings were all too brief and there were many requests for further training opportunities. Although as yet unclear on how, hopefully we might soon be able to co-develop basic training modules, probably in electronic form.

Burmese medical schools use English textbooks but, after graduation, all communication in daily clinical settings takes place in the native language. We agreed that subtitling and cultural adaptations of modules could make information sharing more accessible to all, and the UK psychiatric establishment would undoubtably learn a great deal from the exercise.

Mental Health Awareness Workshop with Buddhist Monks and Nuns

Further meetings through contact networks produced a formal invitation to work with Buddhist monks and nuns on mental health awareness. Once again, this really was only possible through introductions by our Burmese UK-based psychiatrists to interested hosts.

Monks, nuns and village elders have great influence on Burmese society and can be impactful ambassadors for mental well-being. They offer a compassionate and patient approach, backed by the status of 'one who knows' and a philosophy that encompasses how to approach suffering and find a way forward. The senior monks at Shan State Buddhist University were aware that understanding mental illness is an important part of their responsibilities and that Western medical approaches to mental well-being may have some useful contributions to make to improve their ability to fulfil their duties. They explained to us their learning style of lectures and discussions with plenty of time to reflect and meditate.

The chanting of 75 Buddhist monks and nuns at the beginning of our first workshop day was a delightful surprise for the six UK visiting psychiatrists. Our hosts exuded a calm but alert energy as they listened carefully to our descriptions of how we understand mental illness and how we treat it. The Burmese speakers in the UK team told popular Buddhist stories and linked the characters' struggles to mental illnesses, including depression, anxiety, psychosis, acute stress reactions and bereavement. Listening to the responses of the monks and nuns, we were reminded of the value of the reassurance which people can receive by hearing their own cultural stories as routes toward finding a way through troubles.

In the small working groups, we offered evidence-based psychological techniques and exercises on psychosocial support, problem-solving and counselling skills. Together we explored what might work in Myanmar. It was wonderful to hear about their experiences of meditation, mindfulness, chanting and teaching Buddhist philosophy. This was definitely something we learned from, and we reflected upon its potential value in UK practice within the NHS. Our third and final morning together was spent exploring ways to attend to the stigma about mental illness in the community.

Main Themes

The following themes were prominent during our work in all three training areas:

1. Mental illness is common and is treatable with psychosocial techniques as well as medication.
2. Rates of mental illness are high around the world, including Myanmar.
3. Stigma is common and needs to be addressed. Everyone can help.
4. People with mental illness and intellectual disability have human rights and can lead full lives.
5. Mental illness often presents with physical complaints or changes in behaviour or difficulties with faith.
6. Communicating with people who have mental illness and offering simple psychosocial support is therapeutic and appreciated.

What Made This Project So Successful

There were many contributions to this successful work, particularly the welcome by the professionals we worked with in Myanmar, the unstinting commitment and hard work of the UK-based Burmese psychiatrist, the eagerness to learn by participants, as well as the culture of courtesy and friendliness. In this project, I would like to particularly highlight the strength and creativity of the team who worked so well with partners and participants in the training sessions.

Much of the planning and organisation happened between actual visits to Myanmar. The UK team met on many occasions in the UK, and this generated a warm and supportive group with a mixture of skills both clinically and personally. This made us more resourceful and creative, and we all learnt a good deal from each other. We were rarely alone during our time in Myanmar, and we were joined by increasingly large numbers of new colleagues and friends each time we visited. Overall, we worked well together during planning and training sessions and had fun together during breaks.

With our Burmese partners, we pondered on how to make the training sustainable. Almost everyone in Myanmar has a phone and Facebook is very popular, so we managed to keep in contact with many trainees. Nevertheless, we clearly cannot do further work until we develop better digital training resources and reliable means of arranging ongoing communication. Structural changes in training and services will take time. We were hopeful that these would develop, since we had already observed developments in a range of social, academic and economic areas even during the five years that we have been visiting Myanmar. However, the military coup early in 2021 changed all areas of life.

2021 – Everything Changed

The most challenging time for the Myanmar team came with hearing stories from our new colleagues in Myanmar who had become involved in the Civil Disobedience Movement. They were bravely risking their lives, careers and family welfare by standing up to the military regime. Many GPs and psychiatrists working on the front line were also struggling with very distressed people in their care. We hoped that the workshops that had been recorded during our recent visits might be useful to them, and that the regular support sessions we were able to offer online using the WHO Humanitarian mhGAP during early 2021 might make a difference. They told us that there was much comfort in knowing that there were people, and governments, watching and caring about them during this very difficult time.

What UK Visitors Learned

Community Care

People in low-resource settings know a lot about community care. They do it as part of their usual family and community life. Young people often have great respect for elders. For people living together in large families, sharing care is common and helps to support struggling families. Family comes first and duty of care is taken very seriously. We often noticed that people smiled as they sat on tiny chairs at tiny tables lined along the pavements, chatting and taking care of each other. Yes, it gets busy and, yes, this may well change. Poverty is damaging, but I sometimes wonder about the community care going on because caring is a part of everyday life. In the UK we are often cared for by strangers when we are most vulnerable, but in Myanmar it will probably be a relative or someone known to that person.

This community spirit extended to how our work was funded. Our venue was usually gifted, teaching aids were provided by the charity *Mind to Mind Myanmar* and local accommodation was often arranged and provided. Living expenses and outings on days off were funded by volunteers themselves. We reminded ourselves that we have more money than many people in Myanmar might ever dream about, so it seemed right to pay for what we could and support local businesses.

Spiritual Life Is Very Important

In Myanmar, where Buddhism touches all areas of life, kindness, gentleness and care is a felt presence, from the waiter serving food in a restaurant to senior staff taking time to bow in a temple. Watching monks and nuns collect food with grace and gratitude on their early morning walks reveals shop owners donating generously, even though they have little themselves.

World Health Organization (WHO) Opens Doors

The WHO training materials were welcomed. Probably every clinician in the world knows about the WHO and its good standards and standing. Managers and senior authorities, and even non-clinicians, know of WHO. The WHO is rapidly developing ever more useful training packages on a regular basis, and these are free to download.

Evaluations and Feedback Do Matter

Evaluations and feedback after training visits are vital to understand what was helpful as well as demonstrating to authorities that there is value in training doctors and other professionals in the care of people with mental illness. Aside from such formal feedback, we received many messages from participants. One example was an email from a GP recounting that he had diagnosed depression and treated it with psychosocial support, and how his reputation and practice had then greatly increased.

Conclusion and Personal Reflections

I was humbled by our hosts' hospitality, generosity and eagerness to learn. I treasure the many presents given to me by participants and hosts and hope that my small gifts to the people I worked with bring happy memories too. One of my favourite memories is working with a psychiatry trainee in a small group of GPs in Mandalay. I watched as he produced lively discussions in Burmese. I looked around the room and saw similar experiences in eight other groups and felt pleased and moved that we had set up something that meant nearly (another) 80 working clinicians were learning more about mental health and illnesses.

Acknowledgements

This chapter is written as a tribute to Dr Chris Vassilas, a core team member, who died suddenly in April 2018. The tributes and comments from many trainees and new colleagues in Myanmar are a wonderful acknowledgement of his contribution to improvements in mental health care in Myanmar. Our gratitude also goes to the late Dr Myint Oo, Vice President of Myanmar GP Society, who passed away in 2021.

References

1. World Health Organization. WHO mhGAP intervention guide for mental, neurological and substance use disorders in non-specialized health settings: mental health Gap Action Programme (mhGAP). version 2.0 ed. Geneva: World Health Organization; 2016.

2. Nguyen A, Lee C, Schojan M et al. Mental health interventions in Myanmar: a review of the academic and gray literature. Global Mental Health. 2018; 5.

Somaliland: Mental Health Training, Recipient Perspective

Djibril Ibrahim Moussa Handuleh

Background

Somaliland is situated in the Horn of Africa. It has experienced decades of civil unrest, poverty and climate adversity. It became a self-declared independent country in 1991, separate from Somalia.

It is a relatively new country that had a war in 1991 that left much of the country destroyed. It has had many health professionals leave the country and this has led in turn to many diaspora volunteers from the USA, Scandinavia and other countries.

There were some mental health hospitals in Berbera and Hargeisa even before independence but not of good quality. Most Somalilanders even now still go to traditional healers for their mental health care. Mental health is often seen as a spiritual problem.

There is a lot of stigma and misinformation related to people with mental illness. There is a large substance abuse problem. The health system is weak in Somaliland including mental health services. Further, there has been a lack of training in mental health for doctors and nurses and other professions.

Volunteering Support to Somaliland

The Somali diaspora have volunteered consistently to support mental health in terms of resources and visiting experts. This chapter outlines the specific role of the King's College, London Somaliland partnership in training doctors and nurses in mental health[1]. This includes a narrative account delivered in the first person related to my experience as part of the partnership.

The partnership has been an important support in my own professional development and career in becoming a psychiatrist. In 2000, medical schools started to be established in Somaliland. Since then, Kings College, along with the Tropical Health Education Trust (THET) has been supporting the Somaliland health system through face-to-face visits complemented by extensive online support to doctors, nurses, pharmacists and other disciplines.

UK volunteer psychiatrists and nurses came to Somaliland to deliver mental health training and training of trainers each year from 2008[2]. Some of those volunteers for the medical student teaching, who came over in 2008, have stayed involved until now and some are my mentors.

On the first trip there was a diaspora Somaliland psychiatrist. This helped make sure that our culture was appreciated in the training. This training became the model for the subsequent years. Topics such as ethics, human rights and spiritual aspects of mental illness were discussed.

We had specific sessions on mental health in Somaliland and local beliefs in the mental health course for students. There were new teaching methods that I have learned to use now, like role play and interactive teaching methods, as opposed to traditional lectures. I was a medical student in the next year's teaching course in 2009. This inspired me and I learned a lot from this.

In 2010, the team introduced the World Health Organization's Mental Health Intervention Guide (mhGAP) as the undergraduate mental health course. Somaliland became a pioneer country with its incorporation of mhGAP in the undergraduate curriculum and being recognised internationally for this.

We have had some UK volunteers who have spent more extensive periods of time in Somaliland. We had a core trainee who supported us in teaching, examining and helping develop services. Another UK psychiatrist volunteer has spent extensive periods of time in Somaliland and is a visiting professor in Borama. In other ways, the volunteer psychiatrists helped in developing mental health services in both the Somaliland and Puntland regions of Somalia. This happened through the direct supervision and service development initiatives of the former mental health representatives and nurses to set up services. The consultant psychiatrists and the senior psychiatric nurses from the UK developed online training and in-country face-to-face supervision for their Somali colleagues to set up, advocate and run mental health services.

Currently the Borama unit mental health providers continue to receive online and face-to-face training with UK-based psychiatrists. This includes books and other resources donated to the unit which helps evidence-based care for the patients in Somaliland. The UK volunteers have inspired us in our work in hospitals and clinics.

What I Have Learned from Volunteers

Since 2010, I have worked as a psychiatry lecturer, and I also provide mental health care[3]. This work has led to innovative community mental health services in which UK consultant psychiatrists were mentoring the lead mental health teams locally[4].

I initially assisted volunteers in delivering an annual two-week mental health course and now lead on this in Borama. I now support the medical school teaching and training throughout the year.

Another way we have learned from our UK partners has been in our exams in medical school[5]. We learned about written papers and OSCEs (objective structured clinical examinations) and we also learned about different types of examining. The first OSCE exams in mental health took place in 2008 as part of the medical student training course. We were able to share this with other fields of medicine and surgery. I became involved in setting up final year exams in psychiatry and the OSCEs that were part of each medical student's psychiatry course. At the moment, we stress the importance of clinical exams through OSCEs using simulated patients to ensure that our students have not only the knowledge of mental health but also the skills.

This was possible with the generous volunteering role of consultant psychiatrists who delivered exams, some coming for several years. This was one way of addressing the human resources mental health gap by training doctors in rolling out mental health services for those who need it the most. Somalia has high burden on the mental health services where one out of every three people has a severe mental health disorder[6].

These volunteers worked with us. They also listened to us. For example, a big problem we have in Somaliland is Qat or Khat chewing, which causes mental health problems. We have been able to make sure that this is a topic in exams as well as in the medical student teaching. Thanks to the UK volunteers for helping us build the foundations and keep standards at a high level, we are now able to lead on our exams ourselves. Examples of such investment in human resources included direct services for Somali people. This included child and adolescent mental health services in Borama schools[7], and Borama forensic service was the first forensic psychiatry service for Somaliland[8].

There was a one-to-one mentorship scheme in psychiatry which was part of the King's Partnership in which a general practitioner or nurse was matched with a senior psychiatrist or a psychiatry nurse to mentor the Somaliland health care workers. The aim was to empower, support and nurture clinicians and practitioners who had an interest in psychiatry and psychiatry nursing, psychology, occupational therapy or social work. In doing so, they would also be better placed to deliver much needed services.

I have been able to turn to my mentors in the UK for advice and they in turn have helped me publish academic papers and pursue my professional development. UK volunteers have had a great influence on us and our practice. We know they have sacrificed a lot in spending time away from their families and jobs in UK and their benefit to our people is immeasurable.

This has helped us progress our work in inpatient care, community outreaches, prisons and schools, and delivering prenatal mental health services in Somaliland.

Conclusion

UK volunteers have provided much needed and valuable support in Somaliland and Puntland to collaborate in services development in areas like substance misuse and forensic mental health services.

The Somaliland-UK mental health link is dependent on the volunteering spirit of the UK psychiatrists both in teaching and in service development, like the building of the inpatient psychiatry unit in Borama[9] (see Figure 14.1) and the training by the UK psychiatrists of

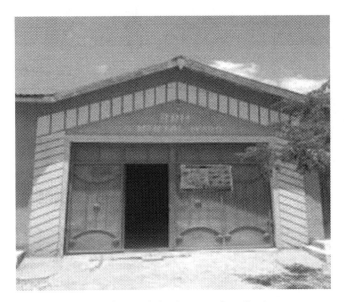

Figure 14.1 Mental health unit which volunteers helped set up in Somaliland

the junior doctors and nurses who were running the mental health facility. The regular online coaching and the in-country visits have helped our staff to deliver competent mental health services. Audits and service improvement initiatives could not have taken place in the setting without the advice from UK volunteers. It helped the international reputation of Somaliland with its pioneering mhGAP undergraduate curriculum.

Somaliland will also need to build research collaboration in mental health which may lead either to fellowships or doctoral training. This would be another area of possible future collaborations with British psychiatrists. At this time, some of us are already specialising and others are on the way to join psychiatry residency programmes to train local psychiatrists.

We are now in a stronger position in Somaliland in mental health and give a big thanks to our UK psychiatry colleagues for helping us to stand on our own feet, but we always will value advice and help in the future from our good friends.

References

1. Leather A, Ismail EA, Ali R et al. Working together to rebuild health care in post-conflict Somaliland. The Lancet. 2006;368(9541):1119–25.

2. Syed Sheriff R, Jenkins R, Bass N et al. Use of interactive teaching techniques to introduce mental health training to medical schools in a resource poor setting: original. African Journal of Psychiatry. 2013;16(4):256–63.

3. Handuleh J. Experiences of a junior doctor establishing mental health services in Somaliland. Intervention. 2012;10(3):274–8.

4. Handuleh JI, Gurgurte AM, Elmi A et al. Mental health services provision in Somaliland. The Lancet Psychiatry. 2014;1 (2):106–8.

5. Sheriff RS, Whitwell S. An innovative approach to integrating mental health into health systems: strengthening activities in Somaliland. Intervention. 2012;10(1):59–65.

6. World Health Organization. mhGAP intervention guide for mental, neurological and substance use disorders in non-specialized health settings: mental health Gap Action Programme (mhGAP). World Health Organization; 2016.

7. Handuleh J, Whitwell S, Fekadu D. Report: school mental health project in Somalia. The Arab Journal of Psychiatry. 2013;44 (473):1–12.

8. Handuleh JI, Mclvor RJ. A novel prison mental health in-reach service in Somaliland: a model for low-income countries? International Psychiatry. 2014;11 (3):61–4.

9. Handuleh J. Transforming a dumping site into a psychiatric inpatient unit in Somalia. American Journal of Psychiatry. 2013;170 (11):1248.

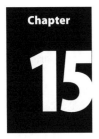

Somaliland and Malawi: Mental Health Training, Trainer Perspective

Mandip Jheeta

Introduction

In 2013, I was fortunate to have the opportunity to teach psychiatry in Boroma, Somaliland for two weeks as part of the King's THET Somaliland Partnership (Tropical Health and Education Trust; KTSP) charitable project. Somaliland is a self-declared independent state and post-conflict area, with a significantly under-developed healthcare system. Mental health is a particularly neglected area. I taught alongside another UK-based psychiatry trainee and project co-lead, with a team of 8–12 Somali co-tutors and staff, including a psychiatry doctor, foundation doctors, senior faculty, nurse and community health workers. We taught and examined 68 medical students. The training was mainly based on the WHO Mental Health GAP Action Programme (mhGAP) manual[1], which is designed to train non-specialists in how to recognise and manage most mental health problems, especially where there is no psychiatrist.

I was also fortunate to teach psychiatry in Malawi in 2015, with the Scotland-Malawi Mental Health Education Project (SMMHEP), for the University of Malawi, College of Medicine. I taught alongside two UK- and three Dutch-based psychiatrists, two of whom were resident in Malawi. It was also partly taught with Malawian tutors, including an associate professor of psychology and medical tutor and a service user representative. I taught 24 medical students for four of their six weeks' intensive psychiatry rotation. In both countries, we used a variety of methods, including interactive lectures, role plays, patient interviews and case discussions. In Malawi, there was additional outpatient 'bedside teaching', film afternoon, and the students ran focus groups exploring mental health views and stigma at a local college. Time was divided between the university and outpatient clinics in Blantyre and Zomba Mental Hospital.

I offer some thoughts on what I learnt from these fascinating and hugely rewarding experiences.

Psychiatry Is Surprisingly Universal

Although I had heard other volunteers give similar accounts, I was still slightly taken aback when first meeting patients and hearing that their descriptions of symptoms and experiences were very similar to what I had heard in the UK. This seemed most true for psychosis, schizophrenia, mania and depression. Indeed, on our first day of students meeting patients, our small group was talking to a gentleman who I had seen briefly in the courtyard beforehand and wondered if he might have negative symptoms of schizophrenia and a mild intellectual disability. To my surprise, 30 minutes later, the gentleman and his mother described exactly these conditions! My experiences emphasised that the fundamental principles of good medical care and teaching are likely to be common across different contexts, that is promoting accurate history taking, examination, investigation, diagnosis, management and developing sound therapeutic relationships. Furthermore, that so much of psychiatry is underpinned by empathy, promoting insight, and investing in trust and rapport with patients and families.

LMICs Medicine Is Often Characterised by Late Presentations, Complex Pathology and Limited Understanding

My colleagues who have worked in low- and middle-income country (LMICs) settings, especially in the emergency department, described how they would commonly see much more complex manifestations of illnesses than we see in the UK; patients seeking help at a much later (and often life-threatening) stage; and local populations often having limited knowledge of various conditions. Indeed, we were told that people with psychotic illnesses in Somaliland commonly first presented to health services after 8–10 years of untreated psychosis. Furthermore, that 20+ years before first presentation is not uncommon. It was also fascinating to hear many first-hand descriptions of catatonia and 'first rank' symptoms of schizophrenia, including several that I had only read about before. In Malawi, we were also told that catatonia (rarely seen in the UK) was commonly seen in the outpatient department until a couple of years ago, when news spread that it could be effectively treated.

Many of the Differences Have Some Similarities, Especially Stigma

Some of the important differences between UK and Somaliland psychiatry involve stigma, khat and suicide. Although also stigmatising in the UK, mental illness is even more and hugely stigmatising in Somaliland, both for patients and families. People with mental illness, particularly psychosis, are often chained and beaten or have stones thrown at them. Even dementia can be stigmatising. Also, psychiatry is often seen as a 'lesser' medical career choice, where professionals must be as 'mad' as their patients! In addition, I had not previously met patients who used khat, an amphetamine-like stimulant. As much of a staple as drinking tea in the UK, chewing khat can lead to psychosis, mania, aggression, and harmful or addictive use. Khat is also commonly used by people to self-medicate their symptoms. Furthermore, suicide in Somaliland mostly affects young women, unlike the UK and global pattern of older men. The main method is self-immolation with kerosene, compared to hanging in the UK and globally. From their professional and personal experiences, our students and co-tutors described how suicide in Somaliland occurs for many diverse reasons, including family and social problems.

Even in these important differences, there were some international similarities – that people with mental illness experience stigma throughout the world; drug use often has a complex relationship with mental illness and can be both the cause and consequence of symptoms; and suicide is a hugely complex issue with no simple explanation.

'Is What I'm Teaching Culturally and Clinically Appropriate?'

Considering differences further, I often found myself questioning if what we were teaching was both culturally and clinically appropriate. Most important, it seems, is to constantly hold this question in mind; and to be inquisitive, adaptable and respectful of the local culture, with a willingness to learn from co-tutors, staff, students, patients and families. In Somaliland, we received excellent locally led sessions on Somali medicine, religion and culture, together with sessions by the service user representative and a multi-faith religious service in Malawi. Basing a lot of our teaching around mhGAP[1] also helped greatly in aiming for our teaching to be international (rather than 'western'), evidence-based, and tailored to resource-limited contexts.

In both countries, I saw how religion, faith and spirituality are interwoven into everyday lives and conversations; and, crucially, into people's ideas about the causes, interventions and treatments for mental illness. For example, in Somaliland, the predominant cause of mental illness is believed to be problems with 'Djinn' or evil spirits, and treatment via the shaikh or spiritual healer is mainly sought first. My experiences taught me to become much more comfortable, interested and confident in acknowledging and exploring faith and spirituality; and to realise that without doing so, something important is likely to be missing from the therapeutic relationship. Indeed, I think discussing spirituality with patients and families is often under-taught and explored in the UK.

As Much About Learning Yourself as Teaching Others

I certainly learnt as much, if not more, than I taught. In Somaliland, I had expected to learn many things about Somali culture, Islam, teaching techniques and medicine and psychiatry in a very different context. However, I did not realise that I would also learn so much about core psychiatry, psychiatric methods and prioritisation. Indeed, very much like in the UK, training has a canny (and at times exposing!) way of revealing 'blind spots' in my own knowledge and skills – and bad habits that I did not realise I had fallen into but was keen not to pass on to the students! It was certainly a two-way learning process.

Decluttering and Focusing as a Trainer

Training in Somaliland, where some students spoke limited English, forced me to think about and become more conscious of ideas and language. Indeed, there seemed to be a constant process of trying to declutter and prioritise. I found it helpful to ask myself 'what is the essence of this idea?' and 'how can I communicate this more precisely?' For example, asking about auditory hallucinations as 'do you hear voices when no one is around?'

I found that less was certainly more. And that it was crucial before a session to be clear in my own mind about what were the few 'take home' messages. Building sessions around key points worked better than covering too much ground. Allied to this, it was important to speak slowly, use repetition, check understanding regularly and be aware that students have a limited attention span.

Even in Malawi and the UK, without a language barrier, decluttering and prioritising ideas, and building sessions around a few key points, remain invaluable skills. Furthermore, the primary overall goal for training is arguably for students to believe: 'Mental illnesses are common and treatable. And I have the confidence, skills and enthusiasm to talk to and help patients and their families.'

Interaction and Variety Are Crucial

I have certainly noticed that sessions work better with more interaction and mixed training methods; for example, a variety of information giving, questions, humour, debate, discussion, quizzes and role play. Whilst I was initially quite nervous about trying more interactive methods, I was surprised at how well they worked. Furthermore, the more I have started to use interactive methods, the harder it is to go back to a more one-way or didactic style. Peter Hughes and Sophie Thomson recommend never using the same training technique for longer than 10 minutes. Whilst I am not yet at this level of skill and creativity, I hope that one day I will be!

I also think that there are other reasons to enjoy and promote an interactive and semi-improvised style of teaching. First, the nature of mental health and stigma means that there must surely be an emphasis on practising clinical skills. Second, it is fascinating to learn from students' questions, challenges and debates, which is central to multiple-way conversations and learning. Indeed, our sessions in Somaliland were hugely enriched and made more enjoyable by the frequent topical contributions and recitations of the shaikh and poet in our class. Last, it is helpful to be able to harness the students' 'buzz' and creativity, to imbue enthusiasm and inquisitiveness for mental health, and open up conversations with patients and families.

How I Changed as a Psychiatrist and Trainer

I came back from Malawi recognising that I had started to develop my own training style and beliefs about what good training looks and feels like. I moved from thinking about 'teaching' to 'training', and that even 'training' was often more about 'facilitating' – that is, something more explicitly and intentionally about mutual learning.

My experiences helped me to be more comfortable and embrace things I did not know as well, for example about culture, religion and weaving spirituality and faith into conversations with patients, families and colleagues. I had not done much team-based teaching before. It was enlightening to see more clearly what does and does not work, and this highlighted my own strengths and weaknesses. For example, I realised that I was able to put a class at ease and get them interacting and discussing, and that I had a helpful eye for detail when writing OSCEs (observed and structured clinical examination) and exam questions. Collaboration also improved my tendency to be over-inclusive, helped me refine and prioritise key learning points, and emphasised the importance of 'ending on a high' before attention wanes.

I also learnt, and then adopted, some of the best training techniques and methods I have ever seen from my co-tutors and students. These included using team-based quizzes and a WHO film about suicide and getting the class to interact with each other whilst having an (unknown to them) good or bad quality written on their back to help explore the experience of stigma. It was also enlightening to do some quick and basic epidemiology by asking every student to briefly write down a case of mental illness or self-harm/suicide that they have seen; then, to categorise, share and discuss with the class, to try to understand local patterns of illness and contributing factors.

After Malawi, I realised that I had developed a training style of trying to be approachable, calm and interactive, with a lot of encouragement by asking questions and facilitating discussions. I also recognised that I felt most comfortable with semi-planned and semi-improvised teaching around a pre-planned framework. I also learnt to be more comfortable thinking on my feet, trying to 'be in the moment' with less worrying about what comes next, and not trying to cram too much in. And, crucially, to have an idea of what you want to say and do but be willing and prepared to ditch it if something better comes along.

Integrating Psychotherapy Ideas into Training

In Malawi, I also started thinking about integrating psychotherapy and clinical practice principles into training – in all three areas one needs to be empathic, non-judgmental and actively invest in putting people at ease. And the resulting sessions can often be very different depending on whether or not a 'safe space' has been created.

Other psychotherapy ideas were also invaluable in fostering positive and collaborative training, especially initially establishing ground rules; managing time; setting boundaries; and using a lot of positive reinforcement, role modelling and encouragement. In both countries, investing time in these techniques reaped dividends in transforming an initially quiet and reserved class hesitant about doing role plays or 'getting it wrong' into a much more open, lively and engaging group several days later. I believe that trying to create a psychologically safe space is crucial in aiming for students generally used to a more didactic teaching style to then participate fully in role plays, and openly discuss hopes, fears and stigma about mental health.

Indeed, one of my most memorable experiences in Malawi was ditching the smaller group lesson plan and remaining quiet whilst the students had a fascinating discussion about their personal, childhood and family beliefs about traditional medicine, the degree to which they believed in it and the dissonance that they often felt when it was frowned upon by their medical colleagues and culture. This discussion highlighted two important aims of 'facilitated curiosity' and 'if you want to go deep, you need a psychologically safe space'.

Bringing Learning back to the UK

The most memorable way I brought learning and inspiration from Somaliland and Malawi was to our local psychiatric medical education programme (MEP) in Solihull. I returned to the UK thinking that we had a very good MEP but that it could be improved. So, I led the running of the programme for 18 months, in a team-based approach, alongside three core trainees and a consultant.

I was inspired to research what makes an effective MEP[2–6] – you need to assess the education needs of members; understand and apply the principles of lifelong medical education; have high audience interaction and participation; have senior involvement and presentation; have regular evaluation of the programme's effectiveness; and create a 'buzz'. This resonated with my experiences abroad, and we set about revamping our sessions by developing a greater variety of presentations, including multidisciplinary guest speakers; producing an appealing 'bulletin' summarising the key learning points of the session; having regular audience feedback sessions; producing structured written and oral feedback for presenters; providing cakes; and including a popular consultant-led 'ten minute training' slot, usually on reflective topics like 'things I wish I'd learnt earlier'.

Central to the changes was asking ourselves a common theme from discussions with senior faculty abroad: *'how can we develop structures, systems and processes that actively encourage the improvement, sustainability and evolution of the education programme?'* We received very positive written and oral satisfaction and effectiveness feedback for the programme. Without the leadership and training experiences developed in Somaliland and Malawi, I would not have had the inspiration, skills and confidence to change and improve our local education programme.

An Inspiring Experience, Invaluable Training and an Honour

It was hugely inspiring and humbling to work with such enthusiastic students, co-tutors, staff, patients and families. Above all, the greatest satisfaction was seeing the students, some of whom had their own apprehensions and misunderstandings of mental illness, grow and transform into a group enthusiastic about and comfortable with people with mental illness:

> The best course ever I took in the time I am in the medical school. The course broke the barrier, fearing of mental illness people, and showed us these patients are the same as our patients of medical illness. The teaching system was amazing.

Anonymous Student Feedback

It's hard to think of other training experiences where it's possible to learn such a huge and diverse amount in a few weeks. Alongside formally 'acting up' as a consultant as a final year registrar, I regard my time in Somaliland and Malawi as being amongst the most formative in my 10+ years of postgraduate training and professional development. It has certainly been my most enjoyable experience of many highlights. As well as improved training, I developed much better skills and appreciation in leadership and cultural adaptability, and how to advocate for more positive views on mental health. I certainly came back as a much better doctor than when I left. They were fascinating, challenging and hugely rewarding experiences, with hopefully more psychiatric volunteering to come in the future. It was truly an honour to have been a small part of such wonderful programmes.

Common Questions Asked

1 Does It Cost a Lot of Money?

The Somaliland trip was fully funded by KTSP, including flights, meals and hotel accommodation. For Malawi, SMMHEP covered £500 towards flights.

2 Was It Dangerous?

For Malawi, no, there is no conflict here. However, there are natural disasters, flooding aggravated by climate change and most risky of all are road traffic accidents. Always wear a seat belt in a car in Malawi and make sure the driver is sober.

For Somaliland, the UK Foreign & Commonwealth Office (FCO) 'advise against all travel to Somalia, including Somaliland', and note threats of terrorism and kidnapping. THET provided very helpful detailed mandatory reading and face-to-face induction which addressed safety and logistics issues, including advice on what to do in a hostage or bombing situation. Some of the security measures in place for volunteers were: having an armed security guard escort you between your hotel and the university every day; being picked up from the airport; a mobile phone provided in-country with emergency contact numbers pre-stored; driving in armed transport; and staying at a nice hotel used by other NGO workers. Trips, for example sightseeing, were prohibited unless authorised by THET.

I was certainly worried beforehand, as were my family and friends. I believe it is important to always hold in mind that you must conduct yourself with respect, politeness and consideration to everyone at all times, and be mindful of local customs and hierarchies.

It is important to always keep yourself and others safe, and to err on the side of caution if in doubt. Ultimately, it is best to listen to the advice given, remember that the risks noted by organisations like FCO and THET are real, and to make sure that you are comfortable with the risks involved.

3 How Did You Get Time Off Work?

I suspect that this may be easier as a trainee than in a substantive post. Health Education West Midlands were hugely supportive. I applied for approximately one-half to two-thirds study leave and the rest as annual leave, which was granted. I would recommend spending time to fill out the study leave application form, and clearly detail the many benefits to training and professional development.

4 Do You Get Time to See the Country?

Due to the security situation in Somaliland, we taught for six out of seven days, with the 'day off' spent planning exams and OSCEs. There was a beautiful, emotional and moving closing ceremony and banquet put on by the university at the end. In Malawi, we taught for five days a week and had the weekends free to explore the country, including Lake Malawi and safaris.

5 Was There Any Negative Reaction?

I was often asked by colleagues *'did you have a nice holiday?'* From my experience, the training is intense and exhausting. The evenings were mainly spent meeting and working with co-tutors to prepare upcoming training. It was certainly much harder than my UK job.

6 What Was the Most Surprising Thing?

That rapport can be surprisingly easy to establish. I think this is because of the huge amount of stigma that people with mental illness face. Politeness, eye contact, showing respect and an effort to meet and greet in the local language goes a long way. One phrase that particularly helped to build rapport was *'waxaan rabaa inan barto af Somali'/'ndimalan-khula Chichewa pangono pangono'* or *'I am trying to learn Somali/Chichewa slowly'*.

In Somaliland, I also found myself copying the students' practice of often placing your hand on a patient whilst talking to them, done only with people of the same gender and usually of a similar generation. It was powerful in putting patients at ease, especially as mental illness is often hugely stigmatising, with the chaining and beating of patients being common. The human touch is so important in clinical care.

7 Did You Ever Feel 'Impostor Syndrome'?

Yes, very often. I think there is something very common, if not universal, in the volunteer experience of feeling like you might be a 'fraud', especially when training in a different culture. I think that a large part of the function of such 'impostor syndrome' is to remind us to stay humble, be willing to learn and be culturally sensitive – and as a way of constantly trying to attune ourselves to our students and their training needs.

Conversely, there is also something hugely 'profession affirming' in being able to build rapport with patients, families and colleagues in another part of the world. And realising that my clinical instinct still worked abroad, for example in being able to recognise dementia in Malawi and guide treatment for epilepsy in Somaliland. Every day I was reminded just how valuable my psychiatric training and clinical experience had been. It hugely increased my appreciation of UK psychiatric training, which really is excellent, especially the explicit emphasis on developing communication, training and leadership skills.

8 'Doctor, isn't this caused by Djinn/evil spirits?' and 'Don't I need to go to the shaikh/traditional healer'?

I think that it's helpful to hold in mind that many people in the world believe that mental illness is caused by evil spirits, not a 'biopsychosocial condition'. Indeed, we are very much in the global minority in the UK. It was also common in both countries that most people do not see a direct conflict between believing in spirits and biomedical illness. They commonly have a pragmatic approach of visiting a nurse or doctor when a spiritual treatment has not worked, and vice versa, and will happily use 'combination treatment'.

How to answer the above question caused a huge amount of debate in both countries. However, I think the best answer, simple and elegant, was by a Somali psychiatrist, Dr Jibril Handuleh: *'You may have a problem with Djinn/evil spirits, and you should see the shaikh for that. But I also think you have a problem with mental illness, and I can help with that'.*

9 What Was the Hardest Thing?

Becoming ill with gastroenteritis during both trips. Being unwell and so far away from home and loved ones felt miserable and lonely. Oral rehydration salts, loperamide, patience and optimism were essential!

10 Did You Have Supervision?

Not formally. I felt very well-supported by the numerous conversations, peer support and reflective discussions with fellow volunteers and co-tutors. However, in retrospect, especially if there isn't a peer network in the country, I think it's wise to have (either back-up or additional) arrangements for perhaps one hour per week telephone supervision with a senior colleague in the UK who has international volunteer experience.

11 Is There Anything That You Would Do Differently?

If possible, take a few days off in the UK before returning to work, though practically this may be difficult. After the mental and physical intensity, stimulation and exhaustion, I found it hard to readjust for the first one or two weeks in my UK job. I probably took a few weeks to get fully back into the swing of things. I am not certain why it took this long, but it is probably a combination of having emotionally invested a lot in the training, personally having quite an intense style of working and objectively it being an intense experience overall.

12 What Are the Most Important Things That You Needed to Hold in Mind?

'Be adaptable and willing to learn'; 'you know more than you think'; and 'is what I am teaching clinically and culturally appropriate?'

13 Any Other Tips?

Always have a copy of *WHO mhGAP*[1] to hand. I'm a huge fan – it means that your training and recommendations are evidence-based, safe and effective. And take other key textbooks to use and then give to local doctors at the end, especially the *British National Formulary (BNF)[7]* (most countries have no equivalent), *Oxford Handbook of Psychiatry[8]*, *Psychiatry P.R.N.[9]* and *Where There Is No Psychiatrist[10]*.

14 Did It Help When Applying for Training and Consultant Posts?

Hugely. I spent a long time in higher training and consultant interviews talking about volunteering experiences and VIPSIG activities. It was particularly helpful in highlighting skills and experience in leadership and management, training, cultural competence and making the most of limited resources. It also seemed to be something genuinely stimulating and different for the interviewers, especially the resulting changes made to the local Solihull medical education programme. The experiences also helped me gain further opportunities, for example clinical and educational supervision accreditation and posts as clinical lecturer and examiner, as a *'Train the Trainers'* tutor and as a MRCPsych question writer.

References

1. World Health Organization. mhGAP intervention guide for mental, neurological and substance use disorders in non-specialized health settings: mental health GAP Action Programme (mhGAP). Version 2.0. World Health Organization; 2016.

2. Ghosh A. Organising an effective continuous medical education session. *J Assoc Phys India* 2008; 56: 533–8.

3. Van Hoof T et al. Improving medical grand rounds: barriers to change. *Conn Med* 2009; 73(9): 545–51.

4. Silver I. Planning the content of psychiatry grand rounds through needs assessments. *CPA Bulletin.* 2002; Jun: 19–20.

5. Silver I. How to make your psychiatry grand rounds more interactive. *CPA Bulletin.* 2002; Apr: 19–21.

6. Watcher B. How to make your medical grand rounds thrive. 2010 [cited 11 Jan 2021]. www.kevinmd.com/blog/2010/01/medical-grand-rounds-thrive.html.

7. Joint Formulary Committee. British National Formulary. 80th ed. London: BMJ Group and Pharmaceutical Press; 2020.

8. Semple D, Smyth R. Oxford Handbook of Psychiatry. 4th ed. Oxford: Oxford University Press; 2019.

9. Stringer S, Church L, Hurn J et al. Psychiatry P.R.N. 2nd ed. Oxford: Oxford University Press; 2020.

10. Patel V, Hanlon C. Where There Is No Psychiatrist. 2nd ed. RCPsych Publications; 2018.

16

Zimbabwe: Diaspora Perspective of Volunteering

Dorcas Gwata

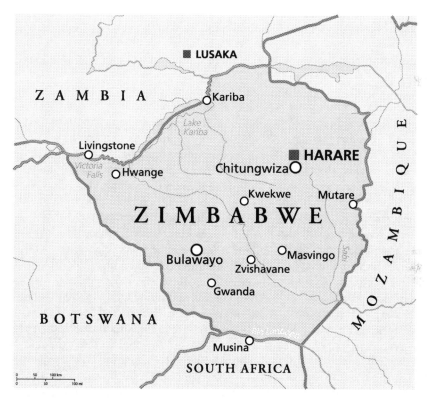

Figure 16.1 Map of Zimbabwe[1]

Introduction

In this chapter, I narrate my experiences of working as a volunteer in my home country of Zimbabwe. I explore the differing challenges and motivations of those of us who have left their homeland to work in the global north and return to volunteer. I finish off by offering 13 tips for volunteering in the continent of Africa.

Getting to Binga Hospital in Zimbabwe

Binga Hospital is relatively small compared to other hospitals we had delivered training and workshops in. The needs here were almost overwhelming for a rural hospital. We had come here at the invitation of Dr Tinashe Goronga, a junior doctor with a huge interest in social medicine and global health.

The desolate road that runs to Binga Hospital in northwest Zimbabwe is long and dusty. There are no western NGOs here, most of them are stationed in the main cities, Harare, and Bulawayo. See Figure 16.1.

Scattered villages give rise to bursting baobab trees, as thin cows scrape the tired grounds for fresh grass. The seasons have been unkind, a ruthless drought and an ailing economy had sunk deep into this impoverished part of Zimbabwe. Women walk the sides of the road, colourful jerrycans of water perched on their elongated necks, babies on their back as drips of water dribble into their eyes.

The occasional rural centre with more bottle stores than supermarkets offers the occasional break from the long drive. We stopped to stretch our legs. The man who served us scanned our TK Max dresses and our fresh long braids, perhaps trying to place us on an invisible map. 'Munobvepi imi ana tete,' he asked of our origins in Shona. That most other tribes in Zimbabwe speak more languages than one, except us the Shonas, was a matter of contention. A bloody history of war, genocide and land grabs had left tensions between the Shona and rest of the country. We were all too aware of the context in which we were coming into this space to deliver training as Zimbabweans living and working in the UK.

In some ways I am home here, my mother's family descended from Zambia into Zimbabwe in the early 1950s long after the British divided the region into slices, taking up most of the fertile lands. My two travel companions, co-trainers and I had taken a week of our holidays to volunteer, giving back to the continent and a country that has birthed, fed and nurtured us to become who we are today. Before we had set off from Harare, Tarisai Bere, my long-term colleague in global mental health, had prepped us on the value of observing local cultures particularly as we were from the diaspora. Of the three of us, Chido, an epidemiologist and PhD student, was more accustomed to the ever-changing turbulences in Zimbabwe. She lived here, so she was less anxious about the currency changes and the cultural expectations of girls and women. Tsitsi and I were easily spooked in the dark, taxi drivers easily ripped us off, we were bothered by the heat and we were known to miss our little comforts available back in London.

Diasporans are sometimes hard to place – we are the ones who left the nest, we live 'abroad', we embody every fibre of culture that symbolises home. We live between two spaces, a spiritual home within, yet home itself is contested. Who belongs and who does not? We find home elsewhere only to miss it deeply, we maintain ties with families and colleagues in health. Home is characterised by remittances, laughter, Afrobeats, loud art, flamboyant weddings, dark and unsettled funerals. The smell of grilled maize-cob, vivacious hair styles and Ankara dresses that sit on wide-hipped women and sometimes men are the very signature of a continent that is as resourceful as it is burdened.

Conscious of our positioning as diasporas coming home to deliver training in a deeply cultural part of the county, we had pre-emptively asked Sister Rena, our mental health contact, for cultural guidance. She advised us not to wear trousers if we were visiting the villages, as being fellow Zimbabweans living away from home this could be perceived as patronising the local culture. She recommended long dresses and covered shoulders when we were training. Sister Rena told us that child marriage and polygamy were common here, some women died in labour and the hospital was away from many villages. We could be curious about the context in which Binga men marry sisters in one family but were told not to patronise or undermine their cultural practices.

She may not have recommended the same to a western visitor who was coming for training session, as 'varungu' white people wear trousers.

Working with Nurses and Doctors

Few trainers venture to these remote parts of the country, the training day is eventful and the team of nurses and administrators attend in their numbers. Sister Rena and the team had gone out of their way to ensure our comfort. The nurses had dressed in their Sunday best, bright African colours and crisp ironed shirts that lit the training room. There was a small issue, which was whispered for ages, the nurses seemed shy. The charity had allocated $2 US to each participant for lunch, the nurses preferred to have the money in cash so they could stretch the money and feed their families, economies of scale.

Over the decades the Zimbabwean economy had tumbled, the country had experienced layers of trauma, the HIV crisis that wreaked havoc in the early 1990s had swept away breadwinners as many migrated within the region and afield. Natural disasters had battered an already ailing population as our politics dug deeper into an abyss. Today more than 500,000 Zimbabweans live in the UK, a good proportion of us work in the healthcare system.

Diasporans are uniquely placed, we come from something, we have a deeper appreciation of the wider context. We are able navigate different contexts under deeply politicised healthcare systems, our lenses are global, yet too often there is little validation or appraisal for the contributions that we make.

Whilst nurses have a good social contract with society, with female nurses making up the core of the workforce, little is understood about the experiences of nurses as breadwinners in society. When the nurses asked for their $2 US allowances in cash instead of bought food, I was aware of the context in which they were making family decisions. Over the tea breaks and during our training sessions we shared our experiences of working in different environments. I talked about my clinical role looking after adolescents who are exposed to gang culture and exploitation in London, and the context of mental health in minority groups in the global north, and they shared their experiences of a deep poverty in Matebeleland and that even though they were struggling to make ends meet, at times they collectively dug into their pockets to collect the bus fare for a patient to get home safely.

I had seen these charitable acts amongst nurses and doctors when I volunteered in India, Tanzania and Myanmar. Some years back, I sat in the mental health ward round in a teaching hospital in Zimbabwe. The junior doctors who led the ward review in some ways were just as vulnerable as the patients they were reviewing. They were not earning much.

As is usually the case, one of the patients had long recovered and was doing well, but he did not have the $6 US equivalent to get back home and there was little social security available. I had encountered the exact same situation in Wedza, where I was a passenger in a minibus that was heading to Marondera. In the distance a poorly woman waved down the minibus, she looked like she might have just been discharged from hospital, her fresh white bandages on her hand gave much away. She leant on her walking stick, as she cleared her chesty cough, she pleaded with the driver, she did not have enough money to cover the fare home, she was short by a $1 US equivalent. I could not bear the suffering, I offered to pay for her and her family to get home. In my clinical years working in global mental health, I had seen the same depth of vulnerability in migrant families who move to the UK in search of safety only to lose their children to gang violence in London. In humanitarian terms the line between clinician and citizenry is blurred. There is a moment in our lives and in the lines of service when our hearts skip, we are torn between deep compassion and sometimes anger.

The world is deeply unequal and it does not apologise for it, and pandemics invariably reveal all.

As a migrant mental health nurse working in the National Health Service, I face layers of discrimination which leave me as a vulnerable as the junior doctors who sat in the ward review that morning. Human suffering is relative, we live in a global village, even in the face of suffering and poverty, there is so much that I take away from low-resourced environments into high-resourced environments. Resilience and innovation live here, volunteering through diaspora lenses brings us that much closer to the experiences of our fellow nurses and doctors working in low-resourced environments.

Facing Gender Issues

In Binga hospital Chido put her research skills to task and led an informal discussion exploring views on sexual and reproductive health with nurses and health care assistants within the hospital. The group engaged well, they generally held strong views on how young girls should behave in society. For instance, it would not be proper or moral for a girl to be seen smoking or drinking alcohol, and sex before marriage was generally unacceptable on the girl's part. We learned more about their narratives, we discussed boys' and young men's responsibility in it all, the group maintained a cultural positioning that generally, men and boys were not expected to behave within the same boundaries as girls.

Collectively as a group of Zimbabweans we began to examine the gendered constraints of our culture in historical and contemporary terms. Our diaspora position brought us that much closer to the narrative than other NGOs might have for instance.

Culture and Migration

I have long been fascinated by the intersectionality between culture, gender, mental health and migration, and volunteering gives that opportunity to converse with communities and health care workers whilst exploring views and perceptions. Some years back I delivered a workshop on global mental health in Myanmar and a similar one in Tanzania. In my workshops, which I often theme 'the grass is not always greener', I usually begin by discussing the realities of nursing in the National Health Service in the UK. I discuss the context in which minority groups are disproportionately over-represented in the mental health and prison systems in the UK and wider western countries. I am all too aware that some of the participants have a glossed-up view of the west, it is not unusual for participants to ask: 'do white people in the west suffer from mental illness like we do in Africa?'

My fellow Zimbabwean Dr Derek Summerfield would have ferociously dived into these kinds of questions, he would have dismantled western perceptions of psychiatry and how it imposes its diagnostics on otherwise culturally explained illnesses[2]. I agree with him to some extent. Summerfield does well in challenging diagnosis, but he does not go further and offer health solutions that lessen the burden. Rather I lean on Professor Vikram Patel's work, 'Where there is no Psychiatrist'[3], and offer the reality that mental health is not purely defined by diagnosis but also by how we access support and if indeed the support is accessible.

Professor Melanie Abas and Professor Dixon Chibanda's work on the Friendship Bench Project[4] resonates, if we take a problem-solving approach and culturally adjusted tools we can provide much relief for those living with anxiety and depression whilst being highly exposed to HIV, domestic violence and substance misuse. The Friendship bench is a literal bench where anyone can sit alongside a trained and wise older person skilled in basic problem-solving skills. But what do we do about gross human rights violations and large institutions that continue to hold 500 plus mental health patients? Here volunteering has its limitations, we have some work to do in the global mental health field.

Hard Realities and Motivations

In global health terms there are stark similarities between a young Black man trying to access mental health care in UK and a young African man who is not able to afford to see the only psychiatrist in the country.

The outcome is the same, they both usually end up being sectioned under the Mental Health Act (or equivalent legislation) and this shapes their experiences of mental health. My view is that it is within the bounds of volunteering to discuss these realities. It is the job of global health to open the world to those who come to learn and share with us. We need a bold leadership that speaks to the truths and acts. Viruses have no borders; mental health knows no race. It is timely then for us examine our conscience, and ask why we choose to volunteer, what are the assumptions that we make when we choose to place ourselves in communities that are less fortunate than us. Are we hoping to change the world? Is our altruism borne out of privilege or a never-ending discomfort of the way the world is? How do we evaluate our interventions and worse still, how do we know when our volunteering efforts are unethical and harmful or not?

The Impact of Volunteering

Covid-19 landed on a bed of inequalities and in the wake of the Black Lives Matter, the debris of uncomfortable global health conversations that was lying on the seabed had been whisked to the surface and we were no longer able to ignore the elephant in the room. The 'white saviour' complex that brings so many volunteers to the African continent for the better or worse must be scrutinised, and the journey of scrutiny begins within. That many of us volunteer is clear. However, we have no true measurement of the impact of volunteering in global health development. The evidence base on diaspora involvement is beginning to gather pace with organisations such as THET, and within my university at the London School of Hygiene and Tropical Medicine, but the research gap remains enormous.

The Well of Resilience

Africa is the birthplace of humanity; it is a vast space with some of the most authentic cultures in our history. In some ways it is unequal to measure its development against the rest of the world. In our altruism we try to fit ourselves into a gap that we perceive to be under-developed and unexposed, yet it is that very well that draws buckets of resilience and innovation within the continent. For the diaspora, our volunteering comes from a deep place of 'giving back' and philanthropy. We need Africa more than they need us. *'Do not thank us, this is God's work,'* nurses and midwives at Chitungwiza often say to me after a training.

It is not unusual for nurses and doctors to pray before or after handover. Indeed, I have always found a greater sense of cohesion and work-life balance in low-resourced environments compared to high-resourced. In the absence of strong structures, health care workers often bond in the common knowledge that all they have is each other. The Muslim community is deeply charitable, the obligation of giving is part of the faith, it is called 'zakat'. The Jewish community comes together in a quiet fashion that is indicative of their history. In African cultures, giving and volunteering is often gendered, women tend to provide care and practical support within communities. There is a lot of cultural and gender capital that is not always visible to the visiting eyes. Many decisions and discussions pass through the matriarchal vein. I have sat in many funeral gatherings and watched grown African men shiver as the matriarchs decide on proceedings.

The balance between vulnerability and resilience must therefore be understood. Whilst many African women may struggle to negotiate the use of condoms to safeguard themselves against HIV and STDs, as well as domestic violence, that vulnerability is not constant, as once empowered they are able to navigate the world in a systematic and governed way, better than those who seek to oppress them. To understand all these dynamics, we as volunteers must be curious and knowledgeable about those we seek to 'save' and help. We achieve this by embedding ourselves in communities, observing dynamics and hierarchies in societies, analysing strengths and weaknesses and viewing the world as a global ecological space. We must think globally and act locally as Lord Nigel Crisp emphasises. He talked of 'turning the world upside down'[5]. We learn from others as much as we give, and we have a common humanity.

Thirteen Tips for Volunteering in Africa (Dorcas Gwata and Tarisai Bere)

1. In order for you to do any work in a new community, it is important to do your research about the people. Learn and understand their ways of living, culture, traditions, language and beliefs. Understand how they describe certain illnesses, for example mental health concepts.
2. Build partnerships with the main gatekeepers (different stakeholders in health), as their buy-in is important for sustainability.
3. Before setting off, take time to make links with the local community.
4. In order not to reinvent the wheel, find out what has been done already. Connect with existing local and diaspora organisations. Observe and learn so that you can fill in the gaps.
5. Build on existing programmes and collaborate with local community leaders and health care professionals, this reduces duplication and conflicts of interests.
6. Check your privilege and motivation for volunteering in Africa, unpack your unconscious bias. Take time to listen as leadership comes from listening and learning.
7. Ethical consideration. Make sure that in whatever you intend to do, you observe good ethical practices as recommended by different institutional review boards. Consider the ethical implications of researching, publishing stories of poverty and poor governance in Africa.
8. Do no harm. Make sure that you protect the rights of the people you work with (partners and participants).
9. Health interventions should be evidence-based.
10. When publishing, consider co-authoring a journal or blog. If given the opportunity to speak about your experience, consider co-presenting with someone who is local, as they own the stories.
11. If you observe human rights violations and safeguarding issues, raise your concerns within the local structures as well as your organisational structures. Human rights are

a global phenomenon, context is important, raise alarm but do not compromise your local partners safety.

12. Capacity building, mentoring and supervision are important for continuity structure and context.

13. Beyond financial ability, ask yourself why you really want to volunteer in Africa and not within your local country where inequalities are significant and concerning.

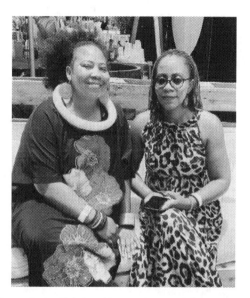

Figure 16.2 Right side is Dorcas Gwata, Global Health Consultant and left side is Tarisai Bere, Clinical Psychologist

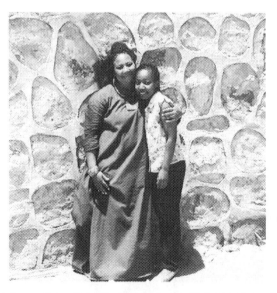

Figure 16.3 Right side is Dorcas Gwata, Global Health Consultant and left side is Tarisai Bere, Clinical Psychologist

References

1. PeterHermesFurian / iStock / Getty Images Plus.

2. Summerfield D. The invention of post-traumatic stress disorder and the social usefulness of a psychiatric category. BMJ. 2001;322(7278):95–8.

3. Patel V, Hanlon C. Where There Is No Psychiatrist: A Mental Health Care Manual. 2nd ed. Cambridge: Royal College of Psychiatrists; 2018.

4. Chibanda D, Mesu P, Kajawu L et al. Problem-solving therapy for depression and common mental disorders in Zimbabwe: piloting a task-shifting primary mental health care intervention in a population with a high prevalence of people living with HIV. BMC Public Health. 2011;11(1):1–10.

5. Crisp N. Turning the World Upside Down: The Search for Global Health in the 21st Century. CRC Press; 2010.

Sierra Leone: Capacity Building, Trainee Perspective on Volunteering

Dawn Harris, and Anna Walder

Introduction

Volunteering in international psychiatry during training has many attractions and advantages. Natural breaks in training occur between foundation, core, higher training and consultant posts and Out of Programme Experiences (OOPEs) have been supported, historically. Many trainees have fewer financial, family and caring commitments earlier in their careers, affording them flexibility to spend extended periods abroad. However, earlier stages of training mean less clinical and management experience and OOPEs need to be balanced between the Royal College of Psychiatrists' regulations about completing examinations and progressing through training. Fortunately, there is a range of opportunities for trainees to get involved, both in-country and remotely, through single one-off placements or repeated visits for shorter durations. In this chapter, we describe one personal experience of long-term volunteering, highlighting learning points and key considerations, as well as indicating alternative opportunities to consider.

Reflections from Volunteering in Sierra Leone by Dr Dawn Harris

In March 2017, I moved to Freetown to volunteer with King's Global Health Partnerships (KGHP) in the role of mental health co-ordinator in Sierra Leone. I stayed for just under 18 months. I had never been to sub-Saharan Africa and did not know anyone else there. I returned having met many exceptional people, with great stories to tell. There were many ups and downs, but it was an incredibly rewarding experience that has shaped my career ever since.

I write this chapter along with colleagues who have previously volunteered with KGPH and have been involved in other global mental health work. Together, we form part of a special interest group called Trainees 4 Global Mental Health, hosted by the Maudsley Training Programme. We hope to increase learning opportunities for trainees in this exciting field. Follow us on Twitter @Trainees4GMH.

Planning the Trip

I had been considering international medical work for many years. During medical school and my early career, I was fortunate to gain general medical experience overseas, but I was unsure whether such opportunities existed in psychiatry. Despite searching, I struggled to find advice about international psychiatry volunteering. I had completed a Diploma in Tropical Medicine and Hygiene at Liverpool University, where the mental health component was limited to just two lectures. Eventually, I found out about the Royal College of Psychiatrists' Volunteer and International Psychiatry Special Interest Group (VIPSIG) and saw the KGHP mental health co-ordination role advertised on its Facebook page. I applied for the position and was later interviewed. In preparation for starting the role I attended a Mental Health Gap Action Programme (mhGAP)[1] orientation weekend, spoke with friends who had been to Sierra Leone and met with KGHP staff for orientation sessions. I was excited to have been offered the post.

Specific Considerations for Trainees

During an approved training programme such as core or higher psychiatry training, UK junior doctors can spend time overseas for Out of Programme Experience (OOPE) or Out of Programme Research (OOPR), such as a studying a master's or PhD or Out of Programme Experience Approved for Training (OOPT). Information about OOPs can be found in the General Medical Council's 'Gold Guide'[2]. Alternatively, junior doctors can take time out during natural career breaks, such as those arising between foundation and core or core and higher training. Advantages of using natural career breaks for international volunteering include increased flexibility and freedom to spend longer overseas. Disadvantages include having to apply remotely for the next stage of training and less certainty about when you will resume clinical training. Other professional colleges have programmes of overseas experiences which fit into their training scheme such as the GP College and South Africa.

Having practised medicine overseas after completing my foundation training, I felt that my contribution to a low- or middle-income setting would be greatest once I had completed my examinations to become a member of the Royal College of Psychiatrists (RCPsych). I travelled to Sierra Leone during a natural career break between core and higher training. Whilst in Sierra Leone I learned a great deal, both from my day-to-day work and through discussions with the UK-based advisory team. This advisory team consisted of global mental health specialists and previous KGHP volunteers. As a trainee, you may only have limited experience in global mental health prior to taking up your position. Pre-employment orientation sessions and having links to an advisory team with experts in the field and local knowledge can be particularly helpful. Some trainees work independently on overseas projects, so creating a supervision structure with space to talk though work with others is useful. See Table 17.1 for considerations related to different voluntary opportunities available.

Time Away

Despite extensive planning (see Table 17.2 for steps needed pre-flight), on the day of my departure, it all suddenly became very real. Whilst I had been very excited about travelling to Sierra Leone, most of my friends and family had been surprised at my choice. Fear of the unknown kicked in at the airport and I remember sitting alone in the departure lounge thinking 'what have I done?' After an anxious flight, I arrived in Sierra Leone during one of the hottest months of the year and was immediately confronted with the heat, a chaotic, crowded airport and a rocky ferry ride to Freetown. However, a warm welcome from my new housemates over dinner helped to settle some of my initial nerves.

Table 17.1 Volunteering opportunities and considerations

Volunteering opportunities	Considerations
Smaller NGOs	Opportunities may be less regular – have to keep checking More responsibility and may have more variety to your role e.g. taking on more administration, funding or grant responsibilities Different supervision and support structures
Larger NGOs e.g. MSF, MDM	May not be available to trainees May require several years' experience, field experience, extra qualifications e.g. membership of RCPsych or languages Can be 'on hold' and have to commit to deploying quickly, thus not suitable for OOP Supportive and extensive training and supervisions structures provided pre-, during and post-deployment
Academic and health partnerships	May have specific requirements for academic or other experience More virtual opportunities May be connections with your current trust or deanery

Table 17.2 Key tasks before you leave

Before you leave	
Administration	Contact the GMC and decide whether to remain on register fully or resign licence. Ideally remain on the register with a licence unless going away for a long period Consider financial implications Consider financial implications including for annual competency review requirements and revalidation (it is feasible, but such processes out of training can be time intensive and expensive) annual competency review requirements (these can be completed though they cost money) RCPsych – full membership required for many opportunities. There may be options to pause steps to examinations OOP requirements, ensure you have prepared all applications for OOPE/OOPT/OOPR in plenty of time – 3 to 6 months in advance
To ask organisation	In-country registration requirements Documents you may need e.g. GMC, university degree Health insurance – what is covered/provided by your organisation? Indemnity insurance Emergency plans Pay/housing/stipend/annual leave/flight allowances
Health	Personal health insurance – is this provided? What is covered/excess amounts? Long-term medication may not be available where you are going, can you get supply, do you need a doctor's letter for arrival customs? Travel health requirements e.g. malaria, vaccinations, Yellow Card
Responsibilities	Is there a defined role and responsibilities? Will there be other volunteers? What handover will you receive? Will it be in-country or pre-departure? Support during the placement, what supervision is provided and by whom?

Freetown Life

Over the following months I adapted to life in Freetown (see Figures 17.1 and 17.2). My accommodation was basic and with intermittent electricity; we were often reliant on generator use. During the rainy season, the sound of the rain on the roof over my bedroom was extremely loud; I slept badly for months. One of my biggest struggles was adjusting to poor internet connection. The house dongle hardly worked. Calls home had to be made from an internet café, with varied quality and privacy. Limited connectivity made being away from family and friends harder. After a few months I began to love living in Freetown, but it took time.

Freetown is located on a spectacular peninsula. I spent many weekends escaping the busy capital and camping on beautiful beaches. Other weekends were spent visiting local markets to buy 'Lappa' (Africana fabric); the local tailor became a regular at our house. An abandoned kitten soon became a loved member of our household and continues to be looked after by one of our housemates now. I also found myself becoming a judge for the Sierra Leone 'Strongest Man' competition at the National Stadium! That night involved many delays and chaotic events, understandably disgruntled contestants, a pitch invasion and a 7am police escort home with two abandoned events.

Sierra Leone and Mental Health

Sierra Leone has a population of approximately 7 million people. In 2017 it had a ranking of 184 on the Human Development Index out of 189 countries, and the shortest life expectancy at 52.2 years[3]. The population has experienced multiple traumatic events including a long

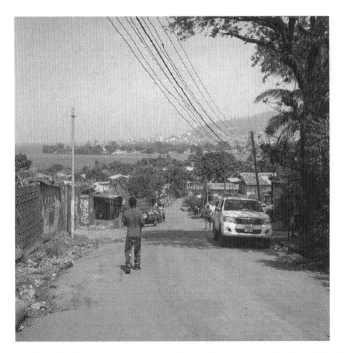

Figure 17.1 Barracks Road, Freetown, the dusty road leading up to our house at the top of the hill with views out to sea

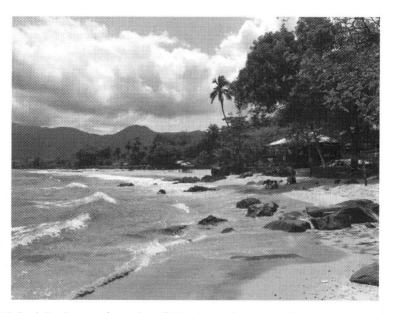

Figure 17.2 Bureh Beach – one of many beautiful beaches on the Freetown Peninsula and the perfect spot for camping at the weekends

civil war (1991–2002) and the 2014–15 Ebola epidemic. In 2017–18 the mental health needs of the population were served by a centralised mental health hospital in the capital, two psychiatrists and 22 mental health nurses mostly operating district mental health units[4]. The treatment gap for severe mental disorders in Sierra Leone has been estimated at 98%[5]. KGHP have been working in Sierra Leone to support the development of mental health services since 2014.

Work Life

My arrival overlapped by two weeks with the outgoing mental health co-ordinator's departure and this handover period was very beneficial in order to get a greater understanding of the project. Along with a second Norwegian mental health volunteer, KGHP worked closely with the national team of mental health nurses. The project aimed to support the mental health needs of Ebola survivors, plus the broader development of mental health services. My role was varied but included supervising the mental health nurses in their clinics, delivering trainings including mhGAP[1], strengthening mental health monitoring and evaluation systems, writing grant reports, plus adapting to any other area of need that arose. Other more unusual activities included going on a march for World Mental Health Day and participating in several radio shows.

Supervising mental health nurses working in local clinics enabled me to travel all around the country and was something I really enjoyed. Initially, I was very aware that Sierra Leonean staff had met new KGHP volunteers every six months. I took time to observe the nurses and understand the setting before feeling confident to give clinical feedback during my visits.

KGHP, in collaboration with other partners, organised quarterly mental health training weeks for the nurses to come together in Freetown. Many worked in isolated rural clinics, so regular meetings were vital for their professional development and morale. The nurses faced a range of challenges that I could never fully appreciate as an international worker, but as we got to know each other, training sessions became increasingly enjoyable and less stressful to organise.

My role also entailed working in close partnership with the Ministry of Health and Sanitation (MOHS) and other partners. I provided technical input to the MOHS as part of the Mental Health Steering Committee and assisted with the development of the national mental health policy and strategic plan. Additionally, we collaborated with the College of Medicine and Allied Health Sciences in Freetown to review the mental health nursing diploma curriculum. This course had not run since its initial conception in 2012 but positively, after supporting the curriculum review, a second cohort of students started training in 2019.

Most people were very friendly and welcoming. Meetings always started with both Christian and Muslim prayers, or with space for silent prayer. Meetings were inclusive, with an opportunity for everyone to contribute, although the complexity and number of departments within larger institutions could be challenging. It was a privilege to work at a ministerial level, from which I learned a great deal.

Clinically, I struggled with seeing patients treated in poor conditions while supervising the nurses. Some patients were chained at home by their relatives or could not afford the treatments they needed. On one occasion, a nurse took me to see a patient in a small town who had been chained up at home for over a year. He was being held in an external shed, with only a rotting foam mattress. The patient was well and had been receiving treatment from the nurse, but she had been unable to persuade his family to unchain him. I was the third international supervisor the nurse had taken to the house to try and persuade the family to unchain him, but they retained concerns about community stigma if he relapsed. We discussed strategies to reduce his risk of relapse and advantages of 'de-chaining'. The family's perspective shifted when I asked when they might feel ready to unchain their relative and in the coming days they did so. Experiences like this made volunteering even more rewarding.

Humanitarian Response Work

One of my biggest challenges came on 14 August 2017 (see Figures 17.3 and 17.4). It had been raining heavily for a few days and district nurses had arrived in Freetown for their quarterly training. By mid-morning, we learned of a large mudslide and flooding on the outskirts of the city, causing over 500 deaths and leaving many people internally displaced. Suddenly, we were thrown into co-ordinating a humanitarian response. The MOHS agreed to deploy the mental health nurses to the affected sites to provide mental health and psychosocial support (MHPSS). We held a meeting that afternoon with local partners and by the next day had deployed the nurses to affected areas, including the mudslide site, flooded villages and regional hospitals.

As well as assisting with the co-ordination of the mental health response, I led a team of nurses deployed at the mudslide site. The survivor support building was noisy and chaotic. It was extremely challenging to provide Psychological First Aid (PFA)[6] in that environment. It was near impossible to link individuals with psychosocial support in the immediate aftermath of the disaster, due to the lack of service infrastructure. The nurses often prayed together with survivors, a hugely important cultural act. We heard tragic stories of sole

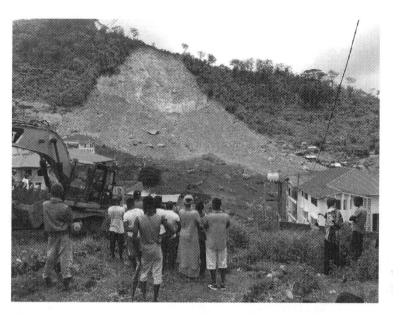

Figure 17.3 Sugar Loaf Mountain on the outskirts of Freetown, site of the 2017 mudslide

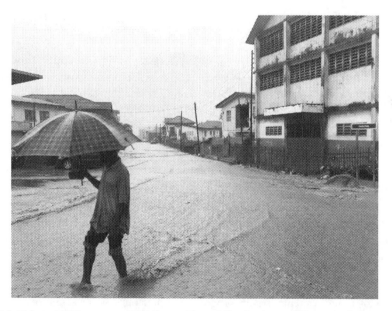

Figure 17.4 14 August 2017 – a man crossing the road through flooding in central Freetown, the same morning as the mudslide and widespread flooding occurred on the outskirts of the city

survivors who had left for work early in the morning and returned to find that their entire family had perished. These accounts were extremely distressing. The tertiary hospital's mortuary quickly reached capacity and empty coffins were piled up in the car park. The work was emotionally and physically exhausting.

Over the following days, internally displaced people were moved to government camps, which soon filled, leaving hundreds to set up unofficial camps, often in large, partially completed houses unfit for human habitation, especially children. Our humanitarian response continued for several months, requiring complete transformation of our working patterns. Learning to adapt and expect the unexpected is one of my abiding lessons from international volunteering. Prior knowledge of PFA was particularly helpful.

When working in low and middle-income counties (LMICs), there may be incidences that you were not expecting, such as floods, landslides, earthquakes or conflict. If you are going as part of a humanitarian response, your organisation would typically give you extensive training on this. However, with smaller NGOs or academic partnerships, this may not be the case. Therefore, it may be helpful to consider whether you would like extra training, for example in PFA, that you could seek to complete yourself. Although you can never prepare for extreme events and your response to them, it could be helpful to talk to previous volunteers and to think of ways you might be able to build both your skill set and resilience.

The Tale of Two Siblings

News of the mental health nurses' work reached local communities over time. In one village, the nurses were asked to see two siblings. They lived in the care of a relative and were struggling with severe untreated mental illness. The siblings were kept locked in their bedroom during the day while their relative went out to beg. They had been abandoned by the rest of their family. Their relative was too afraid to let the siblings outside during the day due to their high vulnerability. They could not cook or look after themselves. They could hardly walk due to limb contractures secondary to immobility.

The nurses assessed both patients, commenced medication and arranged regular follow-up. On my last visit to the family, the KGHP physiotherapist provided advice and exercises to help their contractures and we danced together outside their house. After receiving treatment, both siblings were talking and had started cooking for themselves. They were taking short walks in the village and hoped to reconnect with long-estranged relatives. Seeing their recovery in progress was a highlight of my time in Sierra Leone.

Benefits and Challenges of Longer-Term Volunteering

Relationships

The major benefit of long-term volunteering is the relationships you build with others, in and outside of work. It takes time to build working relationships, especially cross-culturally. Problems were often more complex than they first appeared. At times I thought I understood a problem, only to later discover a misunderstanding that required a whole new approach. Long-term relationships enabled me to get a far better awareness of these challenges and to arrange meetings with key stakeholders to help identify potential solutions. After three and a half years of KGHP's mental health programme, the King's-Sierra Leone partnership was established as one of the leaders in mental health work, with strong links to the MOHS.

My time in Sierra Leone was also made easier by a support network of other long-term KGHP volunteers, who stayed for a year or more. This is not always the norm; many volunteers only stay for six months or less. High volunteer turnover can make it hard to build friendships.

During the period, it is also important to consider how to stay connected with your home country – both professionally and personally (see Table 17.3).

Table 17.3 Connectivity with home country

Staying in touch
• It is important when planning a long-term trip that you have ways and means of remaining in touch with home, for both the personal and the work sides of your experience.
• You may be required to provide blog posts or reports, so check what the rules are and how personal you would like these to be. It may be difficult when you are in the midst of it.
• Consider logging reflections and casework, particularly if you require evidence for annual competency reviews or the GMC.
• If you want to have your own blog, be aware of organisational and confidentiality boundaries, with both writing and photography.
• Keeping in touch with friends and family may be difficult due to lack of connectivity e.g. email and mobile. Think about how you might manage this.
• Contact with past volunteers is a vital resource, providing guidance and understanding of your situation.

Burn Out

Burn out affects many longer-term volunteers. Frustration at unfinished projects and questioning your impact is common. Living, working and socialising with the same people can be claustrophobic. LMICs face extremes of poverty and suffering, alongside stunning natural beauty. Multiple dissonant emotions in the face of so many ups and downs make the experience unsettling. LMICs face a range of challenges, which can easily feel overwhelming so it is important to have your own coping strategies.

Holidays

Holidays are vital to manage the risk of burn out. I went on safari in Kenya and my friends visited me in Sierra Leone. We visited several national parks and some of the many beaches. Daunting moments included canoeing in the dark to a remote island, seeing a cobra slither across the floor of our lodge and traversing puddles the size of small lakes in my 4x4. Our accommodation varied from beach tents to forest cabins and the occasional air-conditioned hotel.

Health

Another consideration for long-term volunteering is your physical health and safety. Roads are dangerous and even the best private medical care is limited. It can be difficult to take prophylaxis regularly; one friend became quite unwell with malaria.

In January 2018 I became unwell with persistent fevers of unknown origin. I was advised to return to the UK for further investigation. KGHP's insurance policy covered such eventualities – a key priority for any prospective volunteer. To my surprise, I was evacuated home on a private medical plane. It was a truly surreal experience (see Figure 17.5).

I could not return to Sierra Leone for nearly a month. It was frustrating knowing that I had limited time left and I wanted to achieve all that I could. The project continued in my absence, my housemates changed, and a new mental health volunteer joined the team. I missed Sierra Leone and could not wait to return. Whilst grateful for the care I received, I reflected on the injustice of spending thousands of pounds on my care, when so little was available in Sierra Leone.

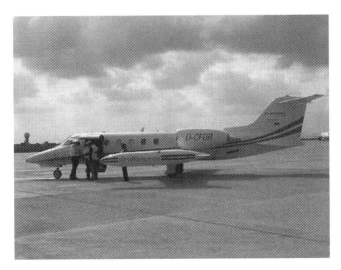

Figure 17.5 Air ambulance plane preparing for departure from Freetown's Lungi International Airport back to the UK

Returning to the UK

Applying for Higher Trainee Jobs

I applied for a higher training position while working in Sierra Leone and had to fly back for the interview. My application was enhanced by my experiences. I had run a national training programme, presented at the Annual Mental Health Conference in Sierra Leone, been first author on a publication highlighting the nursing response to the mudslide[7] and assisted with research projects including one study exploring caregivers perspectives of the child and adolescent mental health service at Ola During Children's Hospital, Freetown.

Leaving

Leaving Sierra Leone was emotional, and I found it difficult to hand over a project in which I was so invested. It was a real privilege to be involved with the MOHS meetings – opportunities I am unlikely to experience in the UK. My mental health work in Sierra Leone will always feel unfinished – there would be no ideal time to leave. I wonder what happened to patients after I left. Did the young man remain unchained? Are the two siblings still receiving treatment?

Coming Home

After 18 months, being home was a culture shock. I missed my lifestyle in Sierra Leone, the weather and visiting beaches at the weekend. I stayed in touch with fellow volunteers and soon wanted to volunteer again.

Workwise, I was accustomed to autonomy and variety, quite different to an inpatient ward. I was so used to the only available treatment options being either haloperidol, chlorpromazine or amitriptyline that I had to brush up on atypicals. The Mental Health Act had changed while I was away, and my peers had progressed into higher training. I appreciated having regular supervision; teaching and academic meetings felt like a great luxury. See Table 17.4 for considerations for return.

Table 17.4 Things to consider on your return

- How can you stay in touch? Some organisations have means for you to remain connected, providing support or supervision to new volunteers. Or providing teaching and supervision online.
- Keeping in contact with friends you made and sharing experiences can also be important.
- How do you keep pursuing global health work at home? It is worth exploring with your supervisor early on when you return, and connecting with others who work in the field.
- Think about how you could develop it during your special interest day. This could be academic (pursuing a master's or PhD), teaching, providing work remotely or working and volunteering for organisations in the UK, for example healthcare for displaced people or medical report writing.

Lessons Learned

If I could repeat my experience, I would make more effort to learn the local language. I lost confidence in learning Krio early on, but many colleagues found it a real advantage in day-to-day life and when teaching.

I learned about grant writing, reporting and liaising with funders. Occasionally, I felt pressured to achieve grant deliverables and to represent my organisation with partners. Some grant deliverables were outside my control. A key learning point is to propose achievable goals when writing grant proposals.

Since returning, I have found it disheartening to learn that the service has struggled with reduced support from international partners. Our KGHP mental health grant finished and there have been limited opportunities for further funding. This is an unfortunate part of development work. The need to plan for long-term sustainability from the outset was one of my key learning points.

There are notable challenges related to volunteering in the time of Covid-19 (see Table 17.5).

Conclusion

Long-term volunteering in Sierra Leone was challenging and extremely rewarding. I had great and difficult experiences and learned a lot about myself. I realised that I could survive without home comforts and I developed a new appreciation for them when I returned. I enhanced my skills as a psychiatrist, with greater cultural awareness and leadership skills. I hope that my work with KGHP in Sierra Leone left a legacy behind, having trained and supported district nurses in mental health skills, and increased prioritisation of mental health care at the MOHS.

As I move forward with my career, global mental health remains a key interest. The work and contacts I developed during this volunteer experience have led me to further opportunities to continue my involvement in this field. Since returning to the UK, I have participated in several research projects, I have presented at an international conference in Ethiopia and I have even undertaken a short teaching trip to Cox Bazar, Bangladesh. I believe that these experiences have enriched and continue to enrich my practice as a psychiatrist in the UK.

Table 17.5 Volunteering in the time of Covid-19

- There have been many changes that will affect trainees who want to work in global mental health and have been considering working abroad. These will no doubt change again over the months and years. There are still long-term projects running that need volunteers, but it is important to consider your health and those around you at home and abroad prior to committing to such a role.
- Increasing numbers of remote working possibilities have arisen and are worth exploring.
- Academic and teaching partnerships require volunteers to provide online courses or assist with teaching.
- There are roles to provide supervision for clinicians abroad or to review clinical documents and policies. There may be health partnerships that your trust or future trusts are connected with that you could become involved with from the UK.
- If you have been considering a diploma, certificate or master's, now may be the time to do it, whilst travelling is still limited.
- There are opportunities to volunteer or work in global mental health in the UK. There may be organisations within your deanery or trust to connect with or NGOs working in your area.
- Keep up to date with research and changes in global mental health and look into organisations that advocate locally.

Acknowledgement

We would like to acknowledge the contributions of Roxanne Keynejad in writing this piece. Your expert technical input and guidance, along with editing skills were vital in the development of this trainee chapter. Thank you.

References

1. World Health Organization. WHO mhGAP Intervention Guide for mental, neurological and substance use disorders in non-specialized health settings. World Health Organization; 2016.

2. General Medical Council. A Reference Guide for Postgraduate Specialty Training in the UK. The Gold Guide Sixth Edition; 2016.

3. UNDP (United Nations Development Programme). Human Development Indices and Indicators. 2018 Statistical Update. United Nations Development Programme; 2018.

4. Harris D, Endale T, Lind UH et al. Mental health in Sierra Leone. BJPsych Int. 2020 Feb 22;17(1):14–16.

5. Alemu W, Funk M, Gakurah T et al. WHO profile on mental health in development (WHO proMIND): Sierra Leone. Geneva: World Health Organization; 2012.

6. World Health Organization, WTF and WVI. Psychological First Aid: Guide for Field Workers. WHO; 2011.

7. Harris D, Wurie A, Baingana F et al. Mental health nurses and disaster response in Sierra Leone. Lancet Global Health. 2018;6(2):e146–7.

Chad, Darfur, Haiti, Sierra Leone and Bangladesh: Humanitarian Field Experiences

Peter Hughes

In this chapter, I reflect upon my experience of volunteering in humanitarian settings across the themes of providing clinical care, non-clinical volunteering activities and specific examples of work (Chad, Darfur, Haiti, Sierra Leone and Bangladesh),. In addition, I reflect on the self-care I have needed in humanitarian contexts.

Clinical Service Provision in Humanitarian Settings

From my own experience, I have provided direct clinical input when there was no one else to do this. In one case, I was invited by a hospital to provide clinical input. This was supported by the government and an NGO. I would only have agreed to do this with this formal host request. It is best to avoid substitution of local workers unless there are none, and there is a clear gap. There may be no health workers due to death, grief, inability to travel to work and sometimes when health workers have managed to escape to a safer place.

Clinically, there may be physical traumatic injury and grief as well as the clinical problems familiar to UK services[1]. A common theme is loss. This may be loss of home, loss of family members, loss of job, loss of status and loss of possessions. Losses can overwhelm, although many people find resources that they didn't know they had, especially if they have family and community support (so called post-traumatic growth)[2]. Religion can also be a great comfort for people. Some however may turn away from religion and this may make them more vulnerable to coping difficulties.

I will now share some examples of cases I recall from times of humanitarian emergency. I can recall seeing a young girl who was depressed because she was about to have her leg amputated and she felt this would make her ugly. Another person with undiagnosed schizophrenia broke his leg in an earthquake and ended up in hospital. He had never been in contact with services before. He had been homeless and destitute. He unexpectedly left the hospital and next I saw him on the street in a wheelchair he had fashioned. He had an external fixator in his leg. He was making good money from begging now that he was clearly disabled to the public. What this reminded me of was people's resilience. They do not need or want to be victims. They are survivors even in the most adverse circumstances.

I have seen many people with what was thought to be clinical depression but was in fact normal grief. It is important not to pathologise grief. This is particularly important in different cultural environments when idioms of distress vary from the UK. I have spent quite a bit of time over the years in humanitarian settings dealing with the effects of grief. This has been some of the rewarding aspects of humanitarian work. In Haiti we supported funerals happening when there was no body through supporting local community religious leaders to have respectful, dignified funerals. Similarly in Sierra Leone during the Ebola time, it was important to support local funerals. At that time funerals were incredibly dangerous due to the risk of contracting Ebola[3]. Our job was to support a safe and dignified funeral that was safe for all attendees. These were times when the role of the psychiatrist expanded significantly.

What I have not seen is many cases of post-traumatic stress disorder (PTSD). When I first went to emergency situations, I learned about PTSD and its management. I expected that my work would revolve around PTSD. What I have found generally is different. I rarely saw any cases of what I could say was clear PTSD and indeed can only think of a few cases. These cases related to victims of kidnapping, sexual violence or car accidents. Almost universally in humanitarian emergencies, people are experiencing stress, but this is entirely understandable and not to be pathologised. The expected figure for PTSD is about 15% in a humanitarian emergency. PTSD can be a somewhat controversial topic. There are those who believe it doesn't exist. There are others who see it everywhere. The answer is likely in between. Fifteen percent is a sizeable number of people. It may not be helpful to give a diagnosis of PTSD to someone if this is not correct as it may lead to sick role behaviour rather than focusing on resilience and building up. Also, in many cases, there is no available specialist treatment for PTSD. So, we are telling people they have a psychiatric disorder and there is no treatment available locally. This may not be helpful. In any case of stress problems or disorder, the principles of stress management are helpful, and psycho-education.What there is no doubt about is the high level of stress and anxiety in any humanitarian emergency.

Non-Clinical Volunteering in Humanitarian Settings

Again, I emphasise the rule for anyone thinking of volunteering in an emergency – do not do it in isolation. Work with a group or organisation that is welcomed by that country. For myself, I have always gone to humanitarian emergencies as part of a responder organisation. In this way, all my needs were met including my accommodation, security and food. It was easy to fit in. Even still, during some emergencies, accommodation was a tent and food was scarce. Security can be a big issue. For example, in the Haiti emergency of 2010 there was a high risk of kidnapping which left us with very restricted movements.

The second rule is to follow international guidelines of IASC (Inter-Agency Standing Committee)[4]. There are some other guidelines for health response called Sphere Guidelines as noted in Chapter 4. These systematically guide all aspects of health and social care and functions to co-ordinate work and be prepared.

Other ways I have been involved were in providing training and capacity building (training health workers) and supporting local leaders and stakeholders in a co-ordinated way. Although it can be an emergency, the humanitarian volunteer can spend a lot of time in meetings with all the people involved, including government representatives. This is actually time well-spent. The government owns and leads on the humanitarian response and the international volunteers need to remember that they are guests.

As a volunteer to some humanitarian emergencies, I can say that it can be a rollercoaster of emotions with fear, frustration, chronic insomnia and discomfort. The pain of dealing with so many in grief is very difficult[4]. On the other hand, there is joy, laughter, fun, friends on a personal level and professionally and the satisfaction of achievement, even for small goals. There are enormous dividends in helping people in the smallest ways. Listening to people's stories when they want to share can be very cathartic for some and validates their experience. The experience of volunteering in a humanitarian setting is very intense. I can recall vividly the humanitarian emergencies in which I assisted. I recall the volunteers for whom this was overwhelming. Some needed repatriation. I knew when it was too much for me and when I needed to have a break. As I write I can recall the smell of the stench of death and unburied bodies, the tears of the bereaved and the loss of a future.

This has been helpful for me to conceptualise PTSD. I can vividly summon up memories of horrible sights but am able to leave them behind thankfully. Being able to shut out these memories in humanitarian emergencies is a necessary skill. Working in humanitarian settings has stretched me like nothing else has. It helps self-discovery and this can be so helpful back in NHS work.

I have learned many lessons myself from my humanitarian emergencies as a psychiatrist:

- Medicines can be used sparingly
- Listening is the most important skill – more important than benzodiazepines and other 'relaxants'
- Your work is beyond being a psychiatrist – you are counsellor, social worker, psychologist, expert on housing, mobile phone technology technician, accountant, practical logistical lead with tents, and many other areas
- It is utterly exhausting
- You have a role to support the people you work with as well
- It can be really hard to adjust back to civilian life and you are in two different worlds for a long time afterwards
- No one can really understand what you went through except those that have been through it themselves
- You can make a real difference
- It brings out the best and the worst in you
- All that we do is about investing in other people
- We know nothing about the countries we go to in terms of their culture and values even when we think we do
- Partnering with local people is crucial and they can be your cultural navigators
- I learned that my psychiatry skills are good but needed to be better for these complex situations
- I learned to keep my work separate from my outside life – immensely useful and transferable to the NHS

Voluntary Placement: Malawi

My first real volunteering experience was in Malawi which I organised independently. This was teaching nurses and medical officers. It was a joy to be in such an immersive experience and learn as much as I was teaching. This was the era of HIV pre–anti-retroviral (ARV) drugs. The horror of seeing so much death from HIV prismed all the teaching around this condition. Subsequent trips to Malawi post ARVs have shown me that things can change, even when you do not think they can at the time. When I returned to Malawi there were people in hospital being treated for conditions other than HIV and they were hopeful of recovery.

It was one of the first times I really understood the importance of culture in manifestation of mental illness. I met people who believed in bewitching and witchcraft. I saw the effect of poverty on people. Malawi remains one of the most enjoyable places I have visited.

Inspired by this, I made contact with some NGOs through the volunteer programme of the Royal College of Psychiatrists which opened doors[5]. Other missions since then have been fortuitous and from word of mouth. After my experience in Malawi[6], I began long-term volunteering connections in Somaliland and Ghana[7].

Voluntary Placement: Chad and Darfur

This arose from the Royal College of Psychiatrists' volunteering scheme. This was my first time working in a refugee camp[8]. I had to get there by joining a United Nations' flight from N'Djamena to the remote eastern region. From our accommodation the refugee camps were an hour's convoy journey away each morning and afternoon with military support. The camps were remote and far from any towns.

It was like another world. There were donkeys everywhere. The only vehicles belonged to the United Nations and NGOs. Otherwise, it was a desert with shelters. Foreigners were not allowed stay at the camps after dark. This was the toughest volunteering experience in terms of day-to-day comforts. There was limited electricity and internet. Sometimes it was a battle against the many large insects which were everywhere. There was no running water. It was a world of water-filled barrels and donkey deliveries. We lived on what was produced locally. There were no real shops. At times security was a problem. Our village had been taken over regularly by opposition and then government forces. We knew that we had an emergency evacuation plan. This was to go to a neighbouring country. Thankfully, I never had to take that up.

Each morning we had a communal meeting with the local community and religious leaders. They would discuss security and health conditions that had arisen overnight. Here, I learned how to treat epilepsy, children's conditions and see face to face the link between poverty, injustice and mental health problems. Epilepsy was seen as demonic or possession but when local people saw that we had good outcomes with medication, word of mouth spread the news and we saw more and more mental health problems of all kinds presenting. Here we worked on dealing with the stigma of mental illness.

I worked with refugee workers who were my cultural navigators. These workers were able to engage with local people. They could go into their homes as they were from that same community. The importance of understanding local culture cannot be under-estimated. From talking to them I got to know a bit about refugee life and their culture. Conditions here were not good and life was hard for all. However, they had strong family bonds and religion was hugely supportive for them.

It was a most extraordinary and inspiring assignment. I can think of my achievements with training and treating epilepsy but probably one of the best things I did was stop antipsychotics being used routinely as calming agents for children. I know the camps are still there and I sometimes think of those I knew still living there in such tough circumstances.

Voluntary Placement: Haiti Earthquake

My mentor in global mental health, Lynne Jones, who has recounted her experiences in a powerful memoir[9], rang me up in January 2010 and asked me to come to Haiti after the catastrophic earthquake. She told me there that there was poor security, lack of food and accommodation. Yet, I couldn't say 'no'. Next, I was in a helicopter landing in an embassy in the destroyed, large capital city of Port-au-Prince, Haiti. The earthquake on 12 January 2010 was shallow and near the capital. The effects were devastating with 220,000 people dead in a short period. Countless people were displaced and wounded.

Port-au-Prince had become a tent city. Hundreds of thousands of people were living in tents or on the street. Early on there were also bodies or body parts on the streets. Next to our base was the nursing school where about 100 nursing students had perished. Everyone I met had a common loss of death, property and livelihood. Every building was a reminder of the death and disaster.

Colleagues from my organisation had arrived within 24 hours of the earthquake. They managed to secure a base for us in a hospital and a residence. We were lucky to have such good support and we never lacked food or shelter. Security was a high priority which was essential in a country with one of the highest kidnapping rates in the world.

Haiti was where I learned most about the bigger picture of working in mental health globally (see Figures 18.1, 18.2 and 18.3). We started with looking at the needs: a situation analysis. We reviewed the previous literature we had on earthquake response. In this case we looked at the Kashmir earthquake of 2005. We also had people with us who had been in previous disasters, including the tsunami of 2004 and could give first-hand accounts. We did not want to substitute any service that was already present so the situation analysis was to look at what was actually still present and what the gaps were.

We followed the principles of the IASC guidelines[4]. This helped frame our response. We ensured that we were working closely with the government who were our hosts. We responded to their requests. We were based at the main hospital in Port-au-Prince (HUEH).

This led to the first strand of work. This was liaison psychiatry in the context of no national people being present at the time to provide this. National staff were deceased, grief stricken or physically unable to get to work with blocked roads, etc. We were able to fill this gap until national staff could take over. We saw people with mental health problems in the hospital.

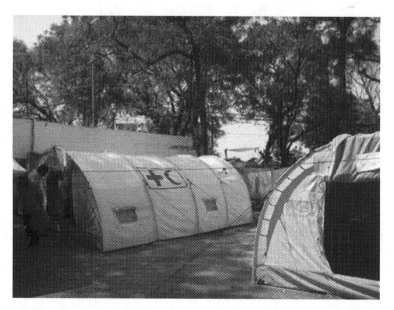

Figures 18.1 Haiti earthquake

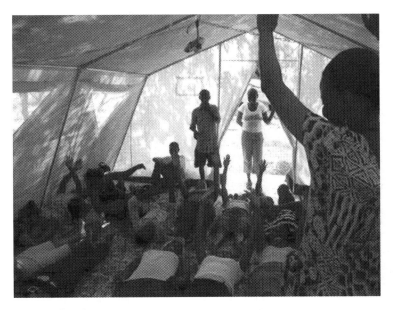

Figures 18.2 Haiti earthquake

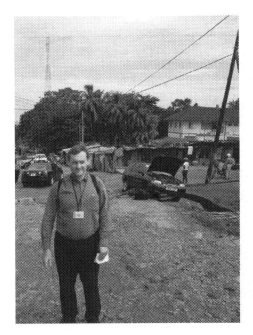

Figure 18.3 Dr Peter Hughes in Haiti

There were people with pre-existing mental illness who had never been treated before in many cases. We saw people with delirium and people struggling to cope with amputations and other physical injuries, as well as being overwhelmed with grief and still not knowing where they would live or how they would earn money when they left hospital. After our work had been completed in the emergency phase, we moved on to a development phase over several months.

People were universally terrified of another earthquake. They preferred to be treated in the tent wards instead of in the main building. This was even when the rats, engorged from feasting on bodies, freely entered. Amongst the many people we saw in Haiti, the commonest problem was palpitations. People feared that they would die or that there would be another earthquake. We rarely used medication. This was all about education and relaxation techniques. As time moved on, we saw less direct earthquake related problems but more of the effects of the stress of living in massive camps, violence and poverty. We started to provide clinics in the different camps once a week. Confidentiality was difficult here when you are under a tree or in a tent separated by a sheet from the rest of the clinic.

Every day, we saw victims of rape. This was awful. We saw so many teenager victims. As a man it was particularly difficult as sometimes there was no female staff member to speak to them. We went through all the protection/safeguarding issues and offered follow-up. What was soul-destroying was that these girls saw it as part of normal life. They knew they would not be able to get justice. Here was a case of giving a lot of listening space and validating their experiences. They would thank me and say it was helpful to talk. I do not know if it was or not, but I always made sure that we would provide them with a tent and a phone to call someone, if nothing else.

We had translators working with us. These translators were hugely important to us as cultural navigators as well as simply translating. I am eternally thankful to my colleague translators, Roro and Fern. They became our friends as well as colleagues. They knew where people came from and about their lives. This filled in the context we needed to treat people properly. Also essential to us were our psychosocial workers who provided the majority of non-pharmacological interventions. In the outpatient clinic as well, we spent a lot of time helping people with their basic needs before anything else. I became an expert on getting tents for people, which was probably one of my more useful roles. Also, we helped people phone their families or get bus tickets to their hometowns. We relied heavily on the principles of Psychological First Aid[8].

We went to the psychiatry hospitals. In one hospital, the walls had collapsed, and many patients had left. Staff were unable to get to work or had their own losses to deal with. We found that the remaining patients had no food or water. This was our task here. We managed to get food and water from the US military. The conditions in the hospital were not good. There were few staff at this time. Emergency clinics were set up in the grounds to deal with the inevitable increase of mental illness that is seen after a disaster.

Here I saw the incongruence of a manic man who had lost much of his family and his house. His son with him had lost a leg. The man was laughing and shouting. There were many families in the grounds sleeping rough. The hospital managed to provide tents for them. It is important to watch out for the most vulnerable. We saw one young girl in a wheelchair. We were able to get help for her from the organisation, Humanity and Inclusion.

As time went on, we saw the mental health conditions in the context of a country that was severally impoverished. The earthquake had just made it so much worse. We went to some remote places that previously had had no services at all. We provided mental health services along with general primary care. I remember particularly the boat clinic which was one hour's speedboat trip from our local base of Petit Goâve. This was an exquisitely beautiful place on the sea only accessible by boat. We saw people with untreated schizophrenia, depression and epilepsy.

Documentation and good records were a priority for us. We knew we were accountable to the government and needed to justify all that we did. Funding finished for our organisation after 18 months. We hoped the government would take over.

One of the main tasks was investing in people and their skills wherever they might be working, so that they could manage mental health conditions on an ongoing basis. My role was teaching, training doctors on the job, setting up primary care mental health services and collecting data.

Thankfully my NHS trust allowed me to step out of my work for a lengthy time for this mission. I thank my mentor Dr Lynne Jones for giving me this opportunity and for her ongoing friendship and support. I also thank the International Medical Corps who sponsored this work.

Voluntary Placement: Sierra Leone

My next emergency mission was working in the Ebola outbreak in Sierra Leone[3]. This was a very different experience as the enemy was invisible now. I learned here about self-care and keeping myself safe. We concentrated on working through standard emergency guidelines on mental health in emergencies with adaptations to local culture and situation. Like Haiti, there was a lot of work on loss. Endless losses.

Here also I learned about paperwork and writing reports. Global mental health work can often be about being stuck in an office, with endless meetings and reports. These actually are important in making a sustainable difference. The main interventions we made here were cascading out Psychological First Aid trainings, staff support and policy development according to IASC. This is important when we consider the nature of ethical support and humanitarian action[10]. The latter meant we needed to look at all levels of health response.

First, people need their basic needs met. Then there is strengthening community supports and self-care. The next level is supporting primary care and secondary care. Responding to all these is important, as is avoiding stand-alone or substitution services. One of the most profound lessons from working here was the importance of people and developing personal relationships.

Voluntary Placement: Bangladesh – Rohingya People

Most recently I have spent some time working with the Rohingya people in Bangladesh[11]. I went to the refugee camps at Cox's Bazar, which is a town close to the Myanmar border. The Rohingya people from Myanmar have been trickling across the border for many years but it has been since 2017 that the mass movement of people occurred in response to the atrocities inflicted on them in the Rakine State in Myanmar. The Myanmar government denies committing genocide.

The camps are cramped, somewhat squalid areas, but seem like bustling towns. The people here are classed as FDMN – Forcibly Displaced Myanmar Nations. This means they lack the usual refugee status. They are not able to leave the camp freely or earn money. They are a conservative people. They speak a type of Bengali/Bangla similar to that spoken in Chittagong, Bangladesh.

I did not have a clinical role here but know that many of the mental health problems were related to stress, psychosomatic problems, suicide and substance use. Generally, PTSD is less common than people might think in such a situation, about 15%. I saw people with substance abuse and suicide. Methamphetamine gets smuggled across the camps (Yabba). This is a particular issue for the neighbouring areas of Bangladesh but also for the refugees.

Psychosis is seen and perinatal problems reported. However, if someone in the camps needs to be admitted to a psychiatric ward, they need to be taken on a 12-hour road journey to the nearest psychiatric unit in Chittagong. The usual treatment is an injection of haloperidol.

There are many organisations in the camps doing great work. The camps are led by the government along with the United Nations High Commission for Refugees (UNHCR) and the International Organization for Migration (IOM). It was important to work well together with partner organisations. There is a lot of psychosocial treatment available with psychologists available. There are very few psychiatrists. When I was there, there was no one with skills in PTSD treatment.

Suicide occurs, particularly in women. This is usually in the context of psychosocial stress. We do not know the figures for the camps but the suicide rate in Bangladesh is unusual in that women are usually at higher risk than men in all age categories. Another important aspect of working in the camps is to ensure that the local Bangladeshi villages have equal benefit of the health care provided for the refugees, otherwise there can be tension. I had to learn a lot about the Rohingya people, not only their history but their beliefs and way of life to be able to work with them on mental health.

Mostly I was office based. Here I was engaged in a lot of trainings and development of the WHO mhGAP programme[12,13]. For me it was training in a training hall mostly away from the camps. Supervision did need to take place at camp level.

The camps were an hour away on some very poor roads. As a volunteer, we always want to be in the field in the middle of the camps with the refugees. However, as a volunteer you must look at where you are most useful. What was satisfying here was to know that the work would continue after I left thanks to all the organisations there.

Other Projects

I have been steadily involved in projects each year. These are usually short-term but the longer-term associations with Sierra Leone and Somaliland have been very satisfying in making sustainable change due to the longer timescale. These have usually been training based.

I have had the privilege of going to some more unfamiliar countries such as Turkmenistan and Afghanistan. There have been many other missions over the years, but I will give another important example of field work – this is being stuck in front of a computer working on papers, reports, online distance supervision and other examples of work that can take place from your home. A lot of volunteering can take place here and is invaluable.

The Covid-19 pandemic has been an opportunity to do online work including training, supervision and staff support. Online work has advantages and disadvantages. For me, it is always preferable to have face-to-face contact, but online contact is undoubtedly more economically sustainable and kinder to the climate.

Self-Care

Humanitarian volunteering includes self-care, which is one of the most important tasks of the global volunteer in challenging settings. I have seen people in humanitarian responses burnt out, broken and unproductive due to overwhelming stress.

Self-care is such an important active task in emergency settings. It is a 'must'. We can only help others if we look after ourselves. We can all reach our burn out threshold. Rest is essential. In humanitarian settings we have a tendency to work all hours and have chronic insomnia. This can lead to habits related to alcohol, smoking or other drugs, eating badly and neglecting exercise. One of my key tasks in humanitarian emergencies is ensuring that all the team are managing their stress and most of all that people utilise their rest. This is important as an individual may feel guilty for taking a break and so, as a team, it is necessary to cultivate a climate to make self-care the norm.

Part of self-care as well is being clear about your job role and goals. Supporting each other is even more important when working in such stressful situations. I can recall many stressful days in the Haiti earthquake time sleeping in tents, but having an evening chat with a colleague was key to me staying well. I realised there though that everyone has their limits and my colleagues had very differing ways of showing their stress when overwhelmed.

Another message that is needed for self-care is that you are not responsible for others. You will hear so many heartbreaking stories. You are asked for money so often, and for jobs. You need to say 'no' and not beat yourself up about it.

I am often asked about danger and how I manage. I really avoid this and make sure wherever I am, I have good security around me. Health wise, I am pretty robust, with the odd case of malaria. The most asked question is, how do I get time off work? This is thanks to sympathetic employers and willing people to cover me over the years.

However, overall, there is always the tension between my work in the NHS, which I love and a deep drive to do global work. There is an uneasy balance that I have had to learn to manage.

Conclusion

I have given a few examples of my work in the short and long term. Key messages from this is the need for humility, to invest in people, understand culture, use evidence base, keep oneself safe and use psychosocial skills. I would urge anyone who is on the point of contemplating some global volunteering to take the plunge. You will not regret it. It will improve your clinical, academic skills as well as your leadership abilities and thinking on your feet. It may well be personally one of the most rewarding things that you can do.

References

1. Rose N, Hughes P, Ali S et al. Integrating mental health into primary health care settings after an emergency: lessons from Haiti. Intervention. 2011;9(3):211–24.

2. Brooks S, Amlot R, Rubin GJ et al. Psychological resilience and post-traumatic growth in disaster-exposed organisations: overview of the literature. Journal of the Royal Army Medical Corps. 2020;166 (1):52–6.

3. Hughes P. Mental illness and health in Sierra Leone affected by Ebola: lessons for health workers. Intervention. 2015;13(1):60–9.

4. Inter-Agency Standing Committee. IASC guidelines on mental health and

psychosocial support in emergency settings. Geneva, Switzerland: IASC; 2006.

5. Royal College of Psychiatrists. Global volunteering scheme of Royal College of Psychiatrists.

6. Scotland-Malawi Mental Health Education Project. Malawi quick guide to mental health. SMMHEP.

7. Syed Sheriff R, Jenkins R, Bass N et al. Use of interactive teaching techniques to introduce mental health training to medical schools in a resource poor setting: original. African Journal of Psychiatry. 2013;16 (4):256–63.

8. Rose N. A working visit to Chad's refugee camps for the people of Western Darfur. International Psychiatry. 2011;8 (1):17–19.

9. Jones L. Outside the Asylum: a Memoir of War, Disaster and Humanitarian Psychiatry. Orion; 2017.

10. Slim H. Humanitarian Action and Ethics. Bloomsbury Publishing; 2018.

11. UN High Commissioner for Refugees. Culture, context and mental health of Rohingya refugees: a review for staff in mental health and psychosocial support programmes for Rohingya refugees; 2018.

12. Hughes P, Thomson S. mhGAP – the global scenario. Progress in Neurology and Psychiatry. 2019;23(4):4–6.

13. World Health Organization. mhGAP intervention guide for mental, neurological and substance use disorders in non-specialized health settings: mental health Gap Action Programme (mhGAP). World Health Organization; 2016.

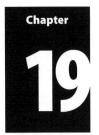

Sudan: Mental Health Training, mhGAP Trainer Perspective

Jane Mounty

Introduction

In 2011 as a consultant psychiatrist, newly retired from the NHS, I decided to apply to the Royal College of Psychiatrists' volunteer scheme to teach in Sudan. On setting out, my biggest fear was failing to meet my contacts at the airport. I knew that once I was linked up with colleagues that all would flow smoothly, and it did!

Sudan is a country which has had a difficult history and accusations of violations of human rights and even genocide. Our team was invited to Sudan just six months before the country split into North and South Sudan. There were deliberations amongst us on the ethical issues about whether it was appropriate to go or not. On balance it was decided that we would go, but as for everywhere we would visit, we would emphasise in our work the human rights of people with mental illness. We would avoid political discussions but follow international principles of human rights.

The Project Development

The training project was developed by the collaborative efforts of the Royal College of Psychiatrists (RCPsych), the Ministries of Health for Sudan and Gezira State and the World Health Organization (WHO) Regional Office for the Eastern Mediterranean. It was also shaped by volunteer psychiatrists from the Royal College of Psychiatrists and others in an international volunteering network, who were recruited as external facilitators.

The project commenced with a 'Training of the Trainers' (ToT) event in Khartoum, where thirty local psychiatrists and psychologists were trained in using WHO mhGAP. The aim was to upscale knowledge of mental, neurological and substance use (MNS) disorders and provide some popular teaching techniques to assist in cascading this knowledge to newly qualified primary healthcare doctors.

For the next seven weeks, in rotation, two volunteer psychiatrists from outside Sudan (UK, Canada, New Zealand, Australia) teamed up with two of the Sudanese facilitators who had completed the Khartoum training and they spent a week teaching groups of around twenty newly qualified family doctors from the University of Gezira in the town of Wad Medani, in Gezira province. The doctors were doing a master's of science in family medicine, so the mhGAP training fitted readily into their programme. Those of us from outside Sudan arrived weekly to join the person who had already covered a week who would then show us the ropes.

I felt privileged to be invited for weeks four and five of this unique experience working alongside mental health professionals who were local as well as from Khartoum. Although each of us international trainers were present for a short time due to the volunteer flow, it actually worked well with continuity. The face-to-face training was followed after a few months by up to one year's online supervision for those family doctors who wanted to develop their skills further.

Impressions of the Country and Its People

I flew via Cairo having never been to Egypt before. Virtually everyone on the connecting flight to Khartoum was in Arab dress and laden with goods. Sudan was the largest country in Africa before the split into North and South. Together, they are vastly ethnically diverse with almost twenty different tribes and one hundred languages. Forty per cent of the people identify as Arab and seventy per cent are Muslim, with five per cent of people identifying as Christian. Temperatures in May/June are often above 40 degrees Celsius and can reach 50 degrees Celsius in July, when we were there. From July to September in Khartoum there is heavy rain preceded by the *haboob* – afternoon storms of red dust which can cut visibility to zero.

Sudanese Colleagues and Family Doctors

From the time I found them waiting to greet me at the airport, my colleagues proved wonderful hosts, driving us over 50 miles in an air-conditioned car to our hotel, The Gezira Club in Wad Medani. The next day they kindly provided a sightseeing tour of this desert city, including the Blue Nile, leisure gardens and, rather surprisingly, a visit to a local Pentecost church which was decorated with beautiful hand-embroidered white tapestries ceiling to floor. Later in the week there was shopping at the nearby souk and wonderful hospitality at the homes of some of my female colleagues' relatives. One thing that we saw was the important social and psychosocial aspect of henna decoration for women, especially for weddings. From the very first evening we met regularly as co-trainers to make plans for our teaching the next day, modifying them to fit local needs, based on feedback from our trainees.

Training Days in the Classroom

The family doctors in training arrived promptly at 8 a.m. on the first day of the working week, Sunday – men and women initially sitting separately in the classroom as is the custom. The men were mostly in white shirts and blue jeans, and the women had brightly coloured matching headscarves, tops and long skirts. We asked our hosts if mixed gender groups were acceptable. They said 'yes' but often the men and women would keep to their own gender. However, it was satisfying to see that both men and women engaged and interacted fully as they gained confidence. There were perhaps three men dressed in black and white with long beards and three women wearing niqabs (face veils) and dressed solely in black. They explained that they belonged to more conservative religious groups.

The sessions were punctuated with breaks for daytime prayers at 11 a.m. and 2 p.m. and occasionally by power cuts when we teachers had to hastily adapt our methods such as postponing or abandoning video and PowerPoint presentations! Demonstration role play illustrating different communication skills and interview techniques (or videos) was fol-lowed by the students performing their own role plays. Our family doctors seemed to enjoy the interactive exercises including daily quizzes on the previous day's learning. They worked in twos or larger groups. We also taught problem-solving. Throughout our time together, each family doctor had access to the course material: copies of the WHO mhGAP manual.

On the first day, all trainees were asked to fill in questionnaires on knowledge and attitude to mental health and provide anonymised vignettes of patients they had seen with mental health problems. These were compared with post-training questionnaires. There were also responses on views about mental health. Some saw mental ill health as a spiritual problem.

Clinical Experiences in a Low Secure Facility and Outpatient Clinic, and Visiting a Traditional Healers' Centre

Thanks to our capable and helpful organisers, Zeinat and others, once each week there was a half-day clinical experience at the locked mental health facility at El-Allab Hospital. There we arranged ourselves in groups of four or five family doctors each with a local psychiatrist or international visitor. We examined patients consented by the psychologist in charge there. The patients were suffering from a variety of conditions including psychoses, delirium, substance misuse and disturbed behaviour. I particularly remember a patient who was a long-distance lorry driver with a paranoid psychosis which had been precipitated by taking amphetamine to stay awake on long journeys – something of an occupational hazard, for anyone attempting to cope in similar circumstances.

As WHO was a partner for this training, local officials from Khartoum came to visit during the second week. I understand that this was one of the first, if not the first, field mhGAP training since its launch in Sudan. We showed them around and explained our objectives: training the family doctors on good mental health, how to use the mhGAP for diagnosis and treatment both in the classroom and outpatient clinic, demonstrating a variety of teaching methods other than didactic and encouraging de-stigmatisation of mental illness in the community[1]. Also, we explained the importance of looking at outcomes by comparing knowledge and attitudes pre- and post-course.

The outpatient clinic attached to a general hospital in town was perhaps the best location for our doctors to find patients with problems similar to those from their family practice: depression, anxiety and somatisation problems. This clinic, however, was extremely busy and note-keeping fairly rudimentary, making it difficult to be able to review the diagnoses and treatments of the longer-term patients, which as a rehabilitation psychiatrist, I usually find is one of the most rewarding challenges.

A fascinating experience for me was the half day spent in the desert visiting a traditional healing centre. This was a village with a mosque, a house for the faqi/sheikh/healer, a compound for camels often given in payment for treatment we were told, and many small shelters where patients resided with their families. There was a chronicity about some of the patients we met, many suffering from long-term psychosis. The atmosphere was that of an asylum or rehabilitation facility. Some patients were more acutely ill with florid psychosis. There were people suffering bipolar illness. It was upsetting to find one or two patients with their arms chained as a means of restraint. They were, nonetheless, allowed to move around accompanied by relatives and to speak freely with us if they wished.

Traditional healers usually serve their communities well, but there have been healers in Sudan known to use unacceptable and inhumane methods such as chains, burning or beating to cure or control illness. National legislation is long-awaited to standardise good practice and eliminate harm[2], as attitudes are changing. Increasingly healers, such as the one we met, are happy to collaborate with a visiting doctor making prescriptions of medication available to the clients alongside the spiritual input that they and their families

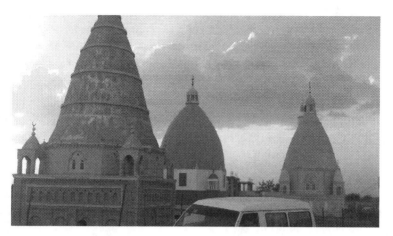

Figure 19.1 Al-Shekaneba in Al-Gezira State. This has a strong heritage in Sufism and is well-known for the traditional and spiritual healing of mental illness

seek[3] (see Figure 19.1). This development and the challenges of human rights for those with mental illness was discussed with the trainees. Some methods of treatment seem strange to our Western eyes.

I recall being inside the mosque where I observed a male patient, part of whose treatment was to drink from a glass of water containing paper with written words from the Koran. Other men present recited prayers over him. Belief in the power of the healer is profound and widely held. During my second week a male student told us in class that his ten-year-old daughter's epilepsy had been cured by the sheikh. Others in the class argued that it was coincidence and 'she had grown out of' childhood epilepsy. In the same week, one of our female students told us that her aim in attending the course was to work alongside her father in his traditional healing practice – providing psychosocial techniques and prescriptions, where beneficial.

Hospitality: Hotels, Food and End of Course Celebrations

There was so much red dust *everywhere* in my first hotel that we needed to be moved to university accommodation and later to a nicer honeymoon hotel (Wad Medina is apparently a popular resort for newly-weds). I gradually realised that the red dust storm, the 'haboob', is an inescapable part of life for all householders and hoteliers at that time of year in Sudan. It also caused my UK colleague's plane to be diverted to Addis Ababa at the beginning of my second week.

Food for us was plentiful; men and women always ate separately. There was a generous breakfast at around 7.30 a.m., lunch at 11 a.m., mainly fried fish or chicken, and an evening meal usually brought to our accommodation. One memorable evening, encouraged by a Sudanese colleague, we took a rickshaw ride around the town in search of *ful medames, a local* speciality. Many times, in the afternoons after class we took Sudanese coffee brewed on the fire and served in a traditional manner.

On the Thursday evening of my first week a magnificent picnic was created for us by our generous students to celebrate the completion of the course. We were invited to the leisure gardens: a vast expanse of green close to the Blue Nile with sideshows and a funfair. The magnificence was in large part created by the beautiful outfits of our hosts: men in full pure white Arab costume, and women dressed in robes of fine cloth with silver and gold thread sparkling in the lantern light of the evening. Their children and babies were also in their best clothes. It felt to me like the set of a film. At first, I had not recognised our resplendent trainees as they ran to meet us across the grass. It was dazzling. We later exchanged gifts: souvenirs of London, biscuits and sweets for our colleagues. For us robes, coffee pots and incense. There was singing and dancing, stories, jokes and laughter. A memorable and magical night. And completely alcohol-free!

Post-Course

The formal post-course assessment measuring changes of attitude, knowledge and skills showed generally positive results and good feedback for the course. These results helped inform each subsequent cohort of teaching.

We revisited the anonymised vignettes provided at the start of the week, asking the students to recommend new solutions for the various biopsychosocial problems described. The cases were mainly psychosomatic problems, depression, epilepsy and social problems, reflecting what patients were bringing to the primary care clinics. Our trainees were very happy to revise the diagnoses described at the start of the week. One patient was diagnosed as suffering from *hysteria* and had been managed by being given *intravenous saline*. It transpired that she was an 18-year-old female student, who the night before an important school exam had presented to her older male GP with severe anxiety and faintness. The family doctors, who no doubt during five or more years of examinations in medical school, had had some similar experiences themselves, now revised the diagnosis to acute anxiety and suggested using psychosocial techniques such as psychoeducation, and relaxation therapy, as they had learned during the training with the mhGAP manual.

Supervision: An Important Yet Challenging Area

Four months after my return, I was invited to participate in a pilot of e-supervision of one of my former students via Skype. In our time together she and I discussed cases from her own practice, involving at least five of the nine mental health conditions in the mhGAP manual. My supervisee particularly wanted support with diagnosis and treatment of her current clinical work. She spent time explaining the cultural context of her patients' problems to me. There were a high number of unemployed patients in her catchment area with a consequent high number of depressed men having problems financially supporting their families. Women locally were usually married at a young age and had large families.

There were two patients with perinatal problems. Both women were under 25 years old with six or more children already, with one suffering from anxiety about how to provide financially for yet another child, and the other suffering prolonged grief over a previous infant death from thalassaemia and fears for the health of her next. As well as discussing depression and perinatal disorders, we also discussed the need for more family planning advice and services locally. Advice was based on guiding the doctor back to the mhGAP manual to find solutions there for any clinical issues.

My supervisee's practice included home visits so as to uncover possible family conflict[4] and to educate the family in understanding the illness, treatment and how best to support their sick relative. Engagement of family in treatment is highly valued, even essential, in the

Sudanese culture. We in the UK might do well to invest more time and effort to adopt similar practices wherever possible and reap the considerable benefits.

From the outset my supervisee found it frustrating that there was little continuity of care because of the way her clinic worked. The patients were seen on a first come first served basis, by whichever doctor was present on the day. The patients too were reluctant to attend for follow-up because of cost and travel issues. The family doctor began negotiating with her seniors for a change in ways of working but, unfortunately, she was not successful in convincing them to change things at that time.

Seven supervision sessions took place over nine months between October 2011 and April 2012 following a format designed by the proposers of the pilot project, based on use of the mhGAP manual. As the authors discuss in their 2015 paper[5], the supervisors training was not standardised and there was a fairly high dropout rate of both supervisees and supervisors. Sadly, some supervisees who had completed all the training and service required of them in Sudan were leaving to start work in wealthier countries due to a range of push and pull factors. The authors also noted that a six-month pilot with one session monthly was not adequate timewise to cover all ten sections of mhGAP.

Discussion, Lessons Learned and Personal Benefits

It was a unique privilege to be invited to participate in the development of another country's mental health services. To gain the trust and elicit the interest and enthusiasm of these young doctors in learning about what in the past had been a stigmatised and unpopular field of medicine was enormously satisfying. Being introduced to the expression of ideas and attitudes toward mental health problems within the Sudanese culture by those most equipped to explain was both fascinating and stimulating. It was a challenge for me personally as a teacher to find ways of enabling the family doctors to add new ways of working to their already considerable skills in treating physical health problems. And above all, realising that despite different cultures and outward appearance, we all have similar mental health problems, stresses and illnesses and these can be understood, diagnosed and managed using the specific step wise evidence-based guidance which makes up mhGAP. It was good to find that mhGAP was readily adopted in the classroom situation and allowed comprehensive cover of nine or ten MNS topics in the relatively short time of five days.

With greater teaching experience and familiarity with mhGAP since then, I realise that in Sudan I could have relied less on PowerPoint, offered more outpatient clinical supervision experience and done a lot more cross-checking with the students. This cross-checking would have been to ensure that they were comfortable with what was being taught but, also, to identify misunderstandings on my part of the culture and beliefs and traditions.

I could have also allocated more time to discussion of ethics and human rights. A further regret was not travelling into the desert after class with one family doctor who begged me to witness in person the very poor conditions in which he found himself working, including no electricity or running water.

After my return, I was inspired to sign up for further studies in anthropology. My experience of teaching in Sudan also proved invaluable in my subsequent volunteer work in the UK with refugees and asylum seekers from all around the world, including Sudan, neighbouring Ethiopia and Eritrea. In 2019 there was another mhGAP training of trainers in Khartoum. This was after the political turmoil of that year. I was told that there were people present from the first training sessions and, although nine years on, it was clear that the previous training sessions in 2011 were the foundations of this further work. I was reassured that sometimes it may take a while, but once the seeds are sewn, progress can continue over time.

References

1. Zolezzi M, Alamri M, Shaar S et al. Stigma associated with mental illness and its treatment in the Arab culture: a systematic review. International Journal of Social Psychiatry. 2018;64(6):597–609.

2. Sorketti E, Zuraida N, Habil M. The traditional belief system in relation to mental health and psychiatric services in Sudan. International Psychiatry. 2012;9(1):18–19.

3. Osman AH, Bakhiet A, Elmusharaf S et al. Sudan's mental health service: challenges and future horizons. BJPsych International. 2020;17(1):17–19.

4. Abdul-Al R. Sources of stress in the practice of psychiatry: perspective from the Arab world. BJPsych International. 2019;16 (3):58–9.

5. Aboaja A, Myles P, Hughes P. Mental health e-supervision for primary care doctors in Sudan using the WHO mhGAP Intervention Guide. BJPsych International. 2015;12(S1):S-16-S-9.

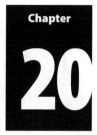

Kashmir: Mental Health Training, Royal College of Psychiatrists' VIPSIG Training Programme

Sally Browning

Arriving in Kashmir

Arriving alone at Srinagar airport, I felt very far from the planning meeting held in London. It seemed an act of faith that I would find my hosts and destination. My faith was rewarded quickly when my two hosts picked me from the passengers at arrivals. Sadly, there are not many European visitors to Kashmir these days, while its political situation remains unresolved. They greeted me warmly and escorted me to a car and driver who would take me to the education centre at Dobiwan, where our course was to be held. On the way there, the driver took a series of phone calls. He informed me that we would have to make a diversion to avoid 'pelting' on our planned route. I had arrived on the day of a demonstration following an incident between the Indian army and local youths. Protesters had lined the roadside of major routes, including ours, ready to pelt with stones any vehicle foolhardy enough to try to pass. We used a disguised vehicle to travel to our residence.

We reached our destination safely but, from this small incident, I had my first intimation of some of the difficulties that face people living and working in Kashmir. None of this sense of surrounding troubles was evident in the hospitality I received on arrival. We were to be looked after by a small team from a local women's charity, HELP. We were treated with immense care by the women of the team, and they were always keen that we should have a chance to appreciate the beauty of their homeland. Kashmir is an exceptionally lovely place with an astonishing landscape (see Figure 20.1). I experienced at first hand the kindness of some of its people in the thoughtfulness and consideration we were shown.

Other colleagues arrived through the rest of the day and, after a welcoming feast of a meal, we held an evening planning meeting with our hosts. As they described some of the logistics of the programme, I began to realise how much planning and organisation had gone into this, from the Kashmiri end of the project.

Preparing to Work

Support had been obtained from all the relevant medical and political leaders and organisations. This had allowed the various permissions required. Importantly, it had allowed the release on study leave of general doctors from every region to attend. Financial backing was obtained from local charities, companies and organisations, including the Kashmiri police who deal with many people with mental health or substance misuse problems. Publicity had been organised and we had an almost daily appearance in local newspapers, which raised our profile and may have raised the status of mental health in Kashmir.

The driving force behind the project was a UK-based Kashmiri psychiatrist Dr Aqeel, who had attended training at the Royal College of Psychiatrists, London and learnt of the

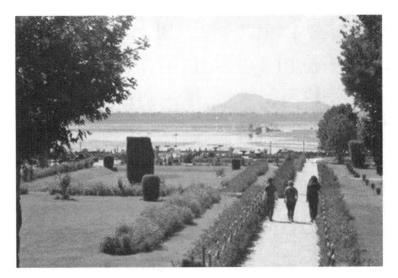

Figure 20.1 Kashmir

Volunteering and International Psychiatry Special Interest Group (VIPSIG) and its training programmes. He began to develop an idea of how such training could be an important part of a plan to develop psychiatric knowledge and practice in his home region and this led to a meeting at the College and an invitation to VIPSIG to deliver training based on the principles of the World Health Organization's (WHO) Mental Health Gap Action Programme (mhGAP)[1].

Initial promotion of the course was by newspaper advertisement, followed by personal contact, using the support of the Director of Health. He was a key individual who allocated doctors and nurses from each of the region's 12 districts, with doctors coming from as far as Ladakh. In all, 40 doctors and 18 nurses were allocated this way.

The target group was those delivering primary care, but other relevant groups also became involved, including a specialist in ayurvedic medicine, social workers, teachers, counsellors, speech therapists, police officers and representatives from supporting NGOs.

Training Days

Our overall teaching structure was laid out from the beginning using mhGAP chapters as a guide, but we made initial modifications following our introductory session. This was a lively and useful meeting with much participation. It gave us a better idea of which subjects were particularly relevant locally and which there was less need for. Further modifications were made as training progressed, based on the daily feedback we received. This enabled us to fine-tune some of the content and develop a style which encouraged participation and was reported as improving learning by the trainees.

We had planned to have two types of small groups – one for prescribers, who were nearly all doctors, and one for non-prescribers. The enthusiasm for training in substance misuse from both types of groups made us decide to undertake this as a plenary session, making use of the knowledge of the local experts available, as well as going through the fundamental issues we had originally planned to teach on.

We met together every evening, both to plan the next day's teaching in more detail and to share reports of each group's experience that day and the issues raised. We used this to influence our planning, so that we could aim to respond to training needs as they were identified, while keeping to the original framework.

That first evening, my co-trainer, Jane, and I discussed our plans for the next day. We had been allocated a group of doctors. This felt reassuringly familiar but, at the same time, we were aware of how little we understood culturally – would it be acceptable to pair men and women together, for example? Discussion with our hosts and our Kashmiri-born team colleague was very helpful as we considered issues such as these. We were also a little nervous about 'the usual' issues: what would our group be like? Would they take part in interactive sessions or be shy? How would we back each other up if one ran out of steam?

In the event, we were delighted to find a knowledgeable and enthusiastic group, very ready to participate and contribute. The structure of our group sessions began with feedback from and recapitulation of the previous day's teaching. We would then make short PowerPoint presentations using mhGAP materials and break into smaller groups for role play and group exercises. Overall, this involved establishing ground rules, energising and engaging the class and modelling and encouraging them to produce case examples from their own experience for discussion within the group. The only physical tools used were the PowerPoint presentations using a projector. This relied on a consistent power supply, so it was useful to have some flexibility and a back-up plan!

As the course progressed, trust deepened within the group and we heard moving accounts of clinical experiences and dilemmas and, sometimes, of a sense of helplessness when faced with mental health problems they had not been trained to deal with. It was very good to see their increasing confidence and hear examples of how they would improve their care, using the knowledge gained.

We also had a few occasions, in private during breaks, when we were asked for advice about family members. This is likely to arise in such a setting and can present a dilemma for trainers who have, on the one hand, a desire to be helpful and supportive and, on the other, a need to maintain the role of educator rather than practitioner. Using relevant mhGAP-based teaching to think through the problems together with the trainee can be helpful, as can the use of fellow trainers for 'supervision'.

Working Together

The plenary session on substance misuse, held in response to demand, was an opportunity to use the expertise of several local participants. It was a specialist area for one of our host organisers, who had much local knowledge to give, beyond the basic framework of guiding principles we provided. One of the student participants was a professor from the medical school, who had taught all the doctors on the course. He was clearly highly respected and his active participation and openness to learning was a very encouraging endorsement to his junior colleagues. The participation of a specialist in ayurvedic medicine was also a very helpful addition to making our discussion locally relevant. The police representative also spoke and was able to give a different perspective in an empathic and compassionate way.

A further plenary at the end of our programme recapitulated some of the basic lessons from the course and acknowledged the value of the support from the various organisations involved. Together, we laid out plans to continue building on the learning and practice developments that had been initiated. Feedback from students was generally very positive and was analysed and, later, produced as a report.

Sustaining the Project

We had planned to continue to support the programme through tutorials following our return to Europe and had arranged access to an internet platform to do this. In practice, this did not work well. The students had to travel to a centre to have access to this and the link kept breaking down, making the process cumbersome and unsatisfactory as a teaching aid. We stopped this, but the local programme has continued and information about progress has been delivered to us regularly.

The programme had mobilised a great deal of enthusiasm from different organisations and at different levels within organisational hierarchies. We had witnessed a collective will to develop better services in mental health for the people of Kashmir. A number of key senior figures involved in training and service organisation had taken part and shown a willingness to take initiatives towards a common goal. Before we left, we and our hosts were honoured to be invited to a dinner with several of them. The discussion there involved initial planning to extend the training from our core group of participants to a wider group of primary care staff and to use this as a means of spreading training across the whole region. To achieve this will require much further work by and cooperation between local stakeholders. We left the meeting hoping that the intervention of our training programme had played some small part as a catalyst, in a situation where there was already acknowledgement of a need and a will to move towards meeting this.

What Did I Learn and Gain Myself?

This was a rewarding teaching experience with a responsive group who seemed to make real gains which would improve their practice. I was impressed by the openness and support of senior staff and the solidarity of various disciplines working together in a common endeavour to improve the mental health of their population.

We had provided a point of contact with a group of health workers who felt isolated from the mainstream due to their political situation. Their pleasure in taking part in an international event was evident. I hope it was also helpful for morale and, through the positive publicity, for the status of mental health services.

I learnt from their ingenuity in making the best use of scarce resources and the solidarity of living in difficult circumstances. From the reports we heard, despite the immense stresses of conflict and uncertainty, patients often have better social support than many of the patients I see in the UK.

While mhGAP demonstrated the consistency of core features of mental illness, I also learnt about local differences in stressors, supports and interpretation.

I had not previously been an advocate of manualised delivery for teaching or services, but I found the mhGAP material on which we based our programme very useful and thought it could be adapted and applied to non-specialist settings at home. It left our students with a tool that they could continue to refer to long after we had returned home.

It felt very important that we went by invitation and that we were there to provide a specific component of a much larger effort organised by local people who understood the issues and structures and were committed to improving services for the population to which they, themselves, belonged.

It was a huge pleasure to be in a beautiful place, with a chance to meet some delightful and admirable people and I'm very grateful to our professional hosts, our domestic hosts, the participants and students for this experience.

References

1. World Health Organization. mhGAP intervention guide for mental, neurological and substance use disorders in non-specialized health settings: mental health Gap Action Programme (mhGAP). World Health Organization; 2016.

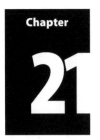

Chapter 21

Ghana: Supervisor Perspective, RCPsych Volunteer Programme

Peter Hughes

Introduction

One of the key tasks for any global training work is supervision. For this reason, I am particularly proud of the Royal College of Psychiatrists and Challenges Worldwide's (NGO) three-month Ghana volunteer programme[1] as we have had supervision with every volunteer since 2007 as well as pre-orientation and debriefing afterwards.

This was a programme created by Sheila Hollins (former College President) and Deji Oyebode (former Chair of RCPsych Volunteering Special Interest Group) through the College of Psychiatrists along with a partner charity, Challenges Worldwide.

The Ghana Project 2007 – Current

Ghana has three psychiatry hospitals and a population of 28 million people. There is a big gap in mental health provision. The psychiatry hospitals are staffed by nurses, clinical officers and doctors. Clinical officers are prescribers who generally have a nursing background with extra training. They are equivalent to the physician associate cadre. They are a key cadre in the provision of health care in Ghana.

The programme involved UK higher specialist trainees in psychiatry spending three months in a hospital in Ghana (see Figures 21.1 and 21.2). Their role was to support staff education and development, particularly the clinical officers. The job had a supervisor in the UK and another in Ghana. A great achievement was having this post approved by the UK Postgraduate Deaneries for three months training. This effectively has opened the doors for valuing the experience of global volunteering for UK training. There was no other similar programme recognised for training in UK. The trainees had an orientation before going and a debrief at the end. During the three months they had weekly distance supervision.

Supervisor's Experience

As the supervisor from the UK, I have had the privilege of overseeing the work of these UK psychiatrists through their three-month rotations since 2007. It has been rewarding to see how each trainee has developed professionally and personally. A project like this brings out the best of people and their resources. I saw this time and time again as these trainees stepped up to the mark with innovative interventions, flexibility and attention to the principles of global mental health. They came back to the UK richer people, personally and professionally. Some were able to conduct research there[2]. Most now work in the NHS as consultants.

In my role as supervisor from a distance, I stepped in more at times and backed off at other times as needed. I interviewed everyone before deployment as part of their orientation

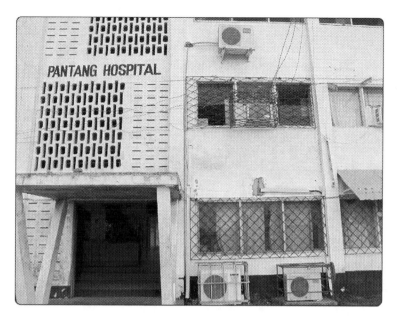

Figure 21.1 Patang Hospital, Ghana

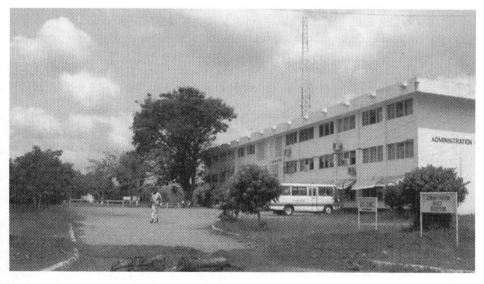

Figure 21.2 Pantang Hospital, Ghana

before travelling and there was a debrief after return. What was essential for me was to have been to Ghana myself and seen the hospitals first hand. I had the privilege of meeting chief psychiatrist Dr Akwasi Osei as well as nurses, clinical officers and other doctors.

The programme evolved with each trainee. Supervision was weekly and based on their weekly report of activity that was e-mailed to me. E-mails to and fro, dependent on internet signal, was the main contact, as well as telephone and Skype support. As supervisor, I would go through every single line of the weekly report and respond. I knew that the internet was not strong and so every single word counted. I recall sometimes I was replying from refugee camps and hoping the internet would work to send a few words.

Sample of Supervision Notes

'In general, clinic should be never with patient and you only but always should be training opportunity with health worker. Job is not service – is training job.'
    'There is no such thing as a patient – it is patient and family. Family almost always know what is wrong.'

We would discuss clinical cases, teaching, research, challenges faced, personal issues and plans for the future after they left. This interactive supervision helped shape the direction of the work led by the trainee. Over time I got to indirectly know the health workers we were supporting in their development, as well as the trainees. Sometimes I was myself in various parts of the world, but the supervision continued without stopping. Each trainee brought something new and changed the programme. The doctors also appreciated a Ghanaian-based supervisor to provide local support.

Trainee Experiences

There were clear phases in the three months of the trainees. The early weeks were a time of adjustment. They needed to settle into their accommodation and deal with practical problems such as finding a bank and machine to get money. There was the culture shock of being in a psychiatric hospital with very different conditions to our own. For the trainees as well as for myself, the first time seeing the wards is difficult if you compare them directly to UK. The staff themselves know that some of the conditions are not good. Some of the wards are overcrowded. There are homeless people abandoned by their families and nowhere to go. Also, what can surprise us is the staff in psychiatric hospitals wearing uniforms and the hierarchies within the staff.

The trainees had different backgrounds and interests. Some had an interest in children while others were more interested in substance abuse, research and transcultural psychiatry. Each person had a different programme that matched their interests, local need and agreed local objectives. There was the opportunity to develop these areas according to the interest of the volunteer psychiatrist. All of the usual conditions that we see in the UK are seen in Ghana. There is a high caseload of substance induced psychosis and schizophrenia in the inpatient units. The outpatients have these as well as anxiety, depression and somatisation disorders. These patients often face the stigma of having a mental disorder in Ghana.

At the early stage, the trainee was often trying to find out what to do and how to do it. It can be an uncertain time. This can be a time of despondency. Homesickness can happen. I am sure that the supervision helped the trainees ground themselves and protect them from burning out. One of the questions we had in selection interviews was 'what would you do if no one turned up for your teaching session?' This did happen not infrequently. Trainees had to learn fast and be flexible. One trainee revitalised breakaway training. Another introduced the mhGAP IG manual[3].

Prayer camps are very important in Ghana, including for those for people with mental illness. Some of the trainees had the opportunity to go and visit these. People with mental illness may be sent to these camps for spiritual treatment. They can be places of hope and support. However, others had violations of human rights. Trainees learned about spiritual aspects and how important this is to people. Skills in mental health advocacy were developed. This is something that can be taken home with them.

The basic skills of history taking, mental state and rational prescribing always needed to be refreshed by each trainee. As a supervisor, I was able to help trainees in the direction of these skills because I had knowledge of the progress of the individual health workers in Ghana over the years.

Having the same supervisor over the years helped the project in many ways but particularly with sustainability. The second half of each three months was about making sure that the benefits of any intervention were sustainable and would continue. By the end of the third month there was usually a rush to get everything done and leave a plan for the next trainee to come over from UK. We tried to have a flow of trainees going over the years to build on our work year on year. Sadly, there have been some problems in organising this more recently. The trainees all valued the experience and felt it helped them in many areas, particularly resource management, leadership and understanding different cultures. Some still continue to volunteer globally.

Learning Points as Supervisor

- Weekly supervision is possible and is useful
- Supervision can be phone, e-mail, Skype – any method of contact
- Long-term sustainability is helped by continuity of supervisor
- Working in low- and middle-income countries in psychiatry can be approved for training
- Trainees even in short periods can produce sustainable change
- It is always important in training globally in mental health to revise the skills of history taking and mental state examination
- Polypharmacy is always an issue
- Stigma is always an issue
- Trainees come back better clinicians and richer human beings after volunteering globally
- Supervision can be very satisfying although it can be demanding as well

Conclusion

As the UK supervisor over the years, I have seen how services have developed and improvements have been sustained. Global mental health and related volunteering is about sustainability and long-term connections. In this case, the supervisor provided continuity over the whole programme, so that each UK trainee could take over seamlessly from the previous one.

References

1. Royal College of Psychiatrists. RCPsych Ghana volunteering scheme. www.rcpsych.ac.uk/news-and-features/blogs/detail/the-rcpsych-blog/2017/04/21/out-of- programme-training-in-pantang-hospital-ghana-dr-konstantinos-tsamakis-april-2017.

2. Poole NA, Crabb J, Osei A et al. Insight, psychosis, and depression in Africa: a

cross-sectional survey from an inpatient unit in Ghana. Transcultural Psychiatry. 2013;50(3):433–41.

3. World Health Organization. mhGAP intervention guide for mental, neurological and substance use disorders in non-specialized health settings: mental health Gap Action Programme (mhGAP). World Health Organization; 2016.

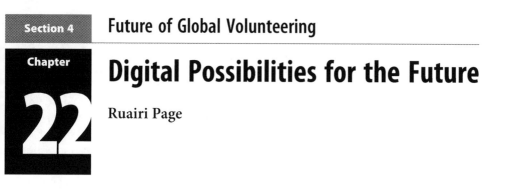

Chapter

Digital Possibilities for the Future

22

Ruairi Page

Introduction

We are fortunate to live in a digital age where technological innovation is progressing faster than ever before. The use of internet-based technology in healthcare and medical education has been forced to evolve at a rate never seen before, as a result of the recent COVID-19 pandemic. Healthcare services are embracing these advancing technologies as they have become increasingly user-acceptable and readily available. These factors, alongside their potential to deliver cost-savings, have resulted in the growth of tele-psychiatry and the delivery of clinical care using technology.

This chapter considers the current use of technology in global volunteering and the future possibilities. Personal accounts and reflections are used at times to illustrate examples of the theories discussed.

Background

Global mental health care and volunteering suffers from a lack of resources, including workforce and financial constraints that impair access to care for many. As such, the technological opportunities for mental health work are immense. The use of electronic technology in international volunteering provides opportunities for the development of working partnerships; an improved and possibly integrated educational approach; research possibilities; the opportunity to build communities of clinical practice; and the evolution of worldwide peer mentoring and supervision schemes.

What Is Happening Now

Training materials are increasingly available online. The World Health Organization's Mental Health Gap Action Programme Intervention guide (mhGAP-IG) is an evidence-based tool aimed at frontline health workers in low- and middle-income countries (LMIC) [1]. It is now available via an electronic format that can be freely downloaded to computers, phones or tablet devices, or used as a mobile App, making it easily accessible by health workers around the globe. These user-friendly approaches used during clinical assessments have been found to be effective[2]. There are also numerous other World Health Organization (WHO) tools and materials including online manuals outlining mental health psychosocial support, group therapy and, most recently, Covid-19 specific online training modules. Notably, there is a new WHO Academy[3]. This is an online global resource to train in mhGAP. Ensuring Quality in Psychological Therapies (EQUIP) is an online platform developed by WHO and UNICEF to support quality in supervision and training in LMICs in healthcare[4]. The Quality Rights toolkit of WHO is available online and is a tool of assessing and improving human rights in health care[5]. This reflects the increasing importance of human rights-based interventions in global health.

Phones and apps increase our ability to communicate quickly and efficiently. We are already witnessing rapidly increasing accessibility to telephone technology and messaging software such as WhatsApp within LMICs. These can produce seamless communication, which is becoming essential in the formation and sustainability of international volunteering projects.

Online learning platforms offer opportunities to engage with cross-cultural education. The very practical and low-bandwidth Medicine Africa[6] is one such tool. An example is the peer-to-peer medical student and nursing global mental health e-learning project, Aqoon, via the Medicine Africa website. This, and other platforms, have been crucial with regard to the development of international volunteering. It has allowed keen volunteers to follow up with the same training cohorts.

Aqoon (Medicine Africa): medical student psychiatric training group facilitation in Somaliland, 2015

The transition between my face-to-face teaching in Somaliland and the facilitation of online-based learning with the same student group was seamless. I found myself teaching in person with the group on a Friday and, after returning to the UK, logging on to Medicine Africa on Sunday to follow up with the group, recap and refresh our clinical skills. We were able to discuss real-life cases concerning people I had met in person at the local psychiatric hospital in Borama, Somaliland. The Medicine Africa platform allowed us to discuss clinical cases easily. There are guidelines on what can be discussed online and it was important for me to follow these. The main joy for me was being able to see the group continue to nurture the psychiatric history, examination and diagnostic skills that we had practised in person, all from the comfort of my own home!

Video conferencing for clinical and other activities is rapidly accelerating, particularly as the Covid-19 pandemic required social distancing and isolation for some health workers. This has resulted in UK mental health NHS trusts developing video conferencing strategies to enable effective communication between multiple sites using simultaneous audio and visual transmission software. Similar approaches have been taken by international non-governmental organisations (NGOs). Subscription to software such as Microsoft Teams, Zoom and others is cheap and readily available in app form, so that it is possible to connect with colleagues from far afield, even from your work car park or garden, should you desire.

These techniques can be used in LMIC settings, provided there is internet and an appropriate platform. It opens up opportunities where there are few psychiatrists for mental health care and for volunteers. This may be particularly relevant given the urban-rural variations in staffing levels in many places.

Clinical activity can also work well electronically, provided the right platform is used

At my NHS trust, a virtual 'Covid-19 medical ward round' using Microsoft Teams was introduced as a way to facilitate overseeing and co-ordinating the medical management of confirmed and suspected Covid-19 patients within our secure psychiatric facility. As a forensic psychiatrist I feel compelled to mention that we have noticed a significant uptake of tele-psychiatry in UK forensic care settings where video technology has actually been used for many years to facilitate distant assessments of patients and for court appearances.

Distance learning is particularly suited to video technology. The use of video technology in remote locations has been well evidenced for many years[7,8], long before the Covid-19 pandemic, and it has been extended to include carer education[9] and supervision of staff [10]. Video technology now helps to develop psychiatric teaching programmes. Key examples from international projects include the use of internet-based video technology for training and e-supervision remotely in Sudan[11], within general practice in remote parts of Australia[12] and the accolades achieved from expansion of remote training programmes for surgical trainees in Scotland[13]. Internet-based training of medical trainees and students using virtual learning environments is also well-established, including in remote areas within high-income countries (HIC) and spanning across the medical and surgical specialties. This has yielded positive outcomes and been very well-received by medical trainees[13]. Blended learning could become the norm for undergraduate training with partial pre-recorded modules complemented by face-to-face seminars.

In the UK, video technology is being increasingly used with successful outcomes in educational programmes, promoting attendance and involvement, whilst also adding a cost-effective benefit in reducing travel time and costs for clinicians. A pertinent example is the development of an educational video conferencing network across forensic mental health services within the West Midlands Forensic Psychiatry Academic Programme (Midlands Partnership NHS Foundation Trust, Birmingham and Solihull Mental Health Foundation Trust) which has now evolved to include renowned international speakers and runs on a weekly basis.

There is a rapid expansion of webinars and other learning opportunities on global mental health from many organisations, including academic institutions and NGOs. They cover a huge range of subjects relevant to volunteers.

Immediate Future Possibilities for International Partnership Working

Many LMICs, in particular those with established universities, medical schools and teaching hospital sites, are now equipped with sufficient internet connection to allow for the same remote learning opportunities as HICs.

So, one may ask, what is stopping students and other healthcare workers around the world from attending the same online-based tutorials that are routinely facilitated in the UK? Of course, the usual limitations would apply, such as a requirement for sufficient bandwidth internet to connect to video-based communication software, time delays, language and cross-cultural issues, cost and ownership of material. But as long as these can be worked around, what is stopping us from inviting colleagues from different continents to teaching sessions which are already being delivered to UK-based colleagues? A simple example would be recording volunteering training sessions, such as the very well-received Royal College of Psychiatrists mhGAP Orientation Training, for those to access at a later date, regardless of where they are located on the planet.

Video networking would also provide opportunities to learn from LMIC colleagues in the future and understand first hand how they develop low-cost and other effective and efficient ways to develop the care of people with mental illness. Perhaps there could be co-production of training packages with colleagues in other countries on topics such as psychosocial support, mental health awareness and cultural adaptation to mental illness.

To aid the implementation of such technological adaptations, it would be beneficial for UK teaching hospitals and NHS trusts to form links or a 'buddy scheme' system with universities or teaching hospitals in LMICs. Tropical Health Education Trust (THET) in the UK has developed a partnership between UK and LMICs institutions. An example is the King's College London-Somaliland project, which has worked hard to develop and sustain a link in mental health training since 2008. The link has gradually moved from pure face-to-face to a blended learning with a strong online presence (see Chapters 14 and 15).

Online training and supervision methods, alongside peer support, could be jointly achieved between colleagues at LMICs and HICs. This would be a truly joint venture of learning, making the most of the advances in digital possibilities. Likewise, the support of network formation and building with digital advances, alongside the development of electronic communities of clinicians, would enable better clinical care worldwide with the sharing of local knowledge to solve local solutions, as well as providing opportunities for shared learning internationally.

Further Forward

Volunteering Networks are already developing amongst the global mental health communities such as THET, Mental Health and Psychosocial Support network and Mental Health Innovation Network (MHIN). The future of international volunteering could one day be to establish a network of volunteers globally. Such an international practice community could, in the future, provide an extended multi-disciplinary opportunity for learning and the peer review of complex and challenging cases or ethical dilemmas, from colleagues from different backgrounds and trainings.

The process of remote partnership working across the international volunteering domain could allow for creative thinking and support across services. This would serve to avoid project isolation and ensure a consistency of approaches to service delivery across diverse services globally. As clinical decision-making carries legal and ethical responsibilities, accountability and other challenges would need to be handled carefully. The use of advancing video technology for international volunteering, and the formation of an international volunteering community, would provide immediate benefits in terms of increased accessibility for training projects, a reduction in the overall training costs and the obvious international travel savings, with a reduced demand in the frequency of face-to-face training, with the added advantage of assisting with climate change. As an example, the World Psychiatry Association is developing a volunteering platform to match volunteer trainers from across the world with institutions requesting training on particular topics[14].

Other fields which are rapidly evolving are the use of virtual reality treatment programmes and online simulation training. These formats are being rolled out locally within the UK at a rate never seen before and for a wide range of uses. These include prominent examples of AVATAR therapy for psychotic patients (initially devised by Julian Leff in 2008 and now trialled successfully by Prof Tom Craig 2020)[15]. This is a technique where people's auditory hallucinations and delusions are conceptualised in a figurative 'avatar' form online. The interaction between patient and avatar is regulated in a therapeutic way to reduce symptomatology. There are other virtual reality software programmes used in psychotherapeutic settings, including within team Balint Groups (Trainee medical psychotherapeutic forum).

An example of online simulation training is for trainee preparation for college examinations. The whole process of medical training examinations in the UK was forced to evolve because of the Covid pandemic. One pertinent example is the Royal College of Psychiatrists' (UK) online version of the CASC (clinical) examination. This is now established and successful. It has enabled candidates to attend from all over the world on an online platform. Online trainee and student examinations may be commonplace in years to come, with the aim of ensuring that the blueprint and structure of examinations remain exactly the same as previously, but with practical examination stations now using online video consultations rather than face-to-face interviews.

Technological developments have transformed our vision of global volunteering for clinical, diagnostic, training and other supports for partnership working. The possibility of remote volunteering within the international sphere also opens up wider research opportunities for colleagues who would have not had these opportunities previously. The future is likely to be computer- or phone-based with our work being largely based on technology. Is this an opportunity to fill the gap of the scarce human capacity resource for the future of global mental health?

What Might This Mean for Face-to-Face Working

With virtual and augmented reality technology progressing at great speed distance volunteering could feel very real indeed. One can do training and supervision that have immersive reality, and this would exceed our current capabilities and meetings could be transformed. The actual distance between volunteer and partner may become transcended as the virtual face to face is close to the actual experience of being in the same room. Virtual reality can be a tool to prepare volunteers for field work and to also test their suitability for the task. Neuroimaging is likely to develop further with capacity to enhance diagnostics online. How this can be further harnessed and translated into helping the global world and volunteering remains to be seen.

Wider societies across the globe are fascinated by artificial intelligence. This has led to the debate about task-shifting away humans in many healthcare roles with technology, even in mental health[16]. Digital technology or 'robots' are now used in many psychiatric healthcare and medical education settings. Whilst it is likely that machines cannot completely take over from the human being, it can be argued that there are a number of areas where the human being has no advantage over the huge capacity of a computer. With certain tasks, computers can work faster and more reliably than us, and amass a much greater amount of information. Computers can be programmed to determine mental health diagnostics, management and even online manualised therapy. We now have face recognition technology with potential capacity to pick up physiological indicators of mental illness. Further, it is now the case, where there is no mental health worker with the right resources, technology may play a role to fill the gap. These technologies are likely to filter to smart phones. It could be that the most useful volunteer of the future is the IT technician who maintains the computer and phone systems. Such technology should not be seen as a lower quality alternative to face-to-face engagement, but instead it could enhance the overall quality, accessibility and affordability of care for all.

Some practitioners may argue that despite the clear benefits that the development of a virtual international community would allow for, including in relation to international peer support, extended peer reviews and network development, artificial intelligence does not take away from the importance and benefits of continued face-to-face working. They may contend that an international virtual community, and the resulting benefits to evolving existing international projects, could only be strengthened with (and not be a replacement for) continued face-to-face training and 'fieldwork'.

There are clear challenges to electronic or 'virtual' working. Many people fear that advances in technology within clinical domains will make us more robotic and dehumanise the holistic nature of our work. The human being must remain at the centre. The technology is to support people, not the other way round. However, we need to accept that technology has advantages sometimes over human workers, and we should embrace this. In mental health, it is not yet clear how artificial intelligence and other technological advances will develop our way of working in global mental health.

Key Points for Volunteering in the Future

- International volunteering is in a major stage of evolution with the development of technology
- We need to be experts in technology and internet
- Virtual technology opens up opportunities to develop and scale up new projects
- There is still no substitute for face to face, this is the gold standard
- Virtual and enhanced reality and simulation may transform our way of working in the future

---

Conclusion

In summary, electronic connectivity technology is now well-developed and well-received worldwide as it has rapidly evolved during the Covid pandemic. There is now a wide range of available video conferencing software to enable seamless video and audio communication across the planet, as long as one has the appropriate internet connection. Both NHS trusts, international NGOs and wider businesses worldwide are reaping the rewards of remote working and internet-based advances, with excellent results and major cost-saving outcomes as a result of new ways of working.

The advantages and benefits of digital conferencing in global psychiatric practice are wide-ranging and make digital communication a priority for the future. A wide variety of mainstream video communication software is now free to use, meaning affordability for all, regardless of where you are on the planet, not to mention the benefits to the environment with digital volunteering meaning that long distance plane travel is no longer essential in all circumstances.

Our international volunteering technological approach to date has been based around using chat-based teaching and supervision programmes for existing projects, such as Medicine Africa. Whilst these have worked well, there are significant compromises in terms of the lack of audio and video communication with the current international training software available. The ideal solution would be to have the same, more evolved, dedicated software programme to be used amongst the global international volunteering domain with easy access for participants, regardless of their organisation, project or location.

The future aims for global mental health volunteering could even include international volunteering academic programmes to involve contributions from renowned worldwide speakers, which could easily be facilitated given the advance in developments with web-based video software. This would allow us all to share the latest in international research with colleagues around the globe, challenge group thinking with regard to international psychiatric research and help recruit volunteers for our new and existing projects at just the click of a button.

Many people in the UK miss the sense of community that face-to-face working brings, and there is no expectation that our colleagues in LMICs will be any different here. What is clear is that developments in electronic working in mental health will continue. How the blend of digital and human work in mental health shapes up in the future is yet to emerge. What that means for volunteering and global mental health may yet surprise us. An opportunity exists for us as global volunteers to shape this space and ensure more accessible, equitable and affordable care is provided for all.

References

1. World Health Organization. mhGAP intervention guide for mental, neurological and substance use disorders in non-specialized health settings: mental health Gap Action Programme (mhGAP). version 2.0 ed. Geneva: World Health Organization; 2016.

2. Keynejad R, Spagnolo J, Thornicroft G. WHO mental health gap action programme (mhGAP) intervention guide: updated systematic review on evidence and impact. Evidence-Based Mental Health. 2021;24(3):124–30.

3 World Health Organization Academy. www.who.int/about/who-academy.

4 EQUIP. www.who.int/teams/mental-health-and-substance-use/treatment-care/equip-ensuring-quality-in-psychological-support.

5 Quality Rights Toolkit. www.who.int/publications/i/item/9789241548410.

6 Medicine Africa. https://medicineafrica.com/.

7. Khalifa N, Saleem Y, Stankard P. The use of telepsychiatry within forensic practice: a literature review on the use of videolink. The Journal of Forensic Psychiatry & Psychology. 2008;19(1):2–13.

8 Curran VR, Fleet L, Pong RW et al. A survey of rural medical education strategies throughout the medical education continuum in Canada. Cahiers de Sociologie et de Démographie Médicales. 2007;47(4):445–68.

9. Haley C, O'Callaghan E, Hill S et al. Telepsychiatry and carer education for schizophrenia. European Psychiatry. 2011;26(5):302–4.

10. Heckner C, Giard A. A comparison of on-site and telepsychiatry supervision. Journal of the American Psychiatric Nurses Association. 2005;11(1):35–8.

11. Aboaja A, Myles P, Hughes P. Mental health e-supervision for primary care doctors in Sudan using the WHO mhGAP Intervention Guide. BJPsych International. 2015;12(S1):S-16-S-9.

12. Greenwood J, Williams R. Continuing professional development for Australian rural psychiatrists by videoconference. Australasian Psychiatry. 2008;16(4):273–6.

13. Smith PJ, Wigmore SJ, Paisley A et al. Distance learning improves attainment of professional milestones in the early years of surgical training. Annals of Surgery. 2013;258(5):838.

14. World Psychiatry Association Volunteering Work Group. www.wpanet.org/wg-on-volunteering.

15. Craig TK, Rus-Calafell M, Ward T et al. AVATAR therapy for auditory verbal hallucinations in people with psychosis: a single-blind, randomised controlled trial. The Lancet Psychiatry. 2018;5(1):31–40.

16. Brown C, Story GW, Mourão-Miranda J et al. Will artificial intelligence eventually replace psychiatrists? The British Journal of Psychiatry. 2021;218(3):131–4.

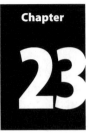

Global Volunteering in Mental Health Moving Forward

Sophie Thomson, Peter Hughes and Sam Gnanapragasam

Global volunteering provides an opportunity to learn, support and work with individuals, communities and colleagues around the world. It can be a hugely rewarding endeavour for all stakeholders if it is undertaken with adequate preparation, developed with host partners and is focused on sustainability. The principles and experiences outlined in this book have sought to provide you with an opportunity to approach the global volunteering placements in mental health with the necessary knowledge, confidence and humility. At the same time, it is important to recognise that much of this book considers how best to navigate the voluntary context as it is here and now. In this chapter, likely changes in the areas of global mental health are presented.

Technology, Remote Working and Virtual Volunteering

Remote partnership working with international colleagues will undoubtedly now expand as electronic learning opportunities increase. It is likely that face-to-face meetings can be blended with electronic opportunities to enhance collaboration on all areas of mental health, including training, service development, academic pursuits, clinical supervision and mentoring. The use of technology offers opportunities to scale up global work to a virtual platform. The increasingly global coverage and use of the internet offers new possibilities for meaningful mental health interventions that offer more regular and sustained contact, as well as having ecological advantages for climate control with less need for air travel.

The Covid-19 pandemic accelerated these virtual voluntary opportunities and placements as outlined in Chapter 22. Now, in the post-Covid era, we can reflect on what will work best for future volunteering. Many would argue that face-to-face work is always far superior, but we have now learned how to incorporate online working. A hybrid model of volunteering appears to be the most likely future way of working. There is a need to properly evaluate the effectiveness of different types of service and training delivery modalities and the use of different types of technology with respect to voluntary projects. Discussions with people currently delivering training and recipients of training suggest that one hybrid model that seems effective is as follows: during an introductory phase prior to face-to-face work volunteers can provide support in planning and offer suggested reading or other learning. This is followed by a period in-country to deliver training in workshop and seminar format. This can be then followed up by remote ongoing supervision by volunteers on return to their home country.

With the growing emphasis on exploring new models of learning and training through virtual hubs, individuals from different parts of the world can concurrently learn together and share experiences. Although this has yet to fully take off across many mental health domains, the potential to pool knowledge and resources (for example, specialist trainer knowledge and skills), as well as promoting cross-cultural learning, has significant strengths. An example is the new WHO Academy[1] where there is an opportunity to learn virtually on a range of health topics. EQUIP (Ensuring Quality in Psychological Support)[2] is also a recent WHO and UNICEF online initiative to assure quality in training and service delivery in mental health .

Further, the way in which care is delivered in both high- and low-income countries may change and, as such, approaches and training may need to be adapted accordingly. It is possible there may be a growing divide in care delivery approaches with accelerated use of technology and tele-psychiatry in one context compared to the other. On the other hand, both contexts may accelerate use of technology at the same time thereby bridging the delivery gap. This will have a direct impact on the skills required, and the content of voluntary endeavours.

Demographic Changes

All countries around the world are undergoing demographic changes, and this will have ramifications for the needs and health profile of nations. This in turn will directly impact on the services and skills that health systems will need to cater for. This will vary significantly between different countries and regions, with some having an older demographic, such as the UK, and others having a largely working age or young population. As such, the mental health conditions that need attention and management may well change and the volunteers' skills and knowledge will need to respond to emerging and changing needs.

Development of South-South Volunteering

There are many diverse models of international volunteering. At present, much of the volunteering is that of North-South volunteering. This means the 'rich Global North' volunteering in the 'impoverished poor Global South'. It is likely that there will be growth and diversity of practices in international volunteering whereby South-South volunteering becomes the predominant feature of global mental health. This means that local countries can help each other without the traditional power imbalance. This will offer opportunities for translation and adaptation of carefully costed innovation, training and service delivery. Volunteers from the United Kingdom and other high-income countries will need to continue to approach the voluntary experience with humility and an appetite to learn and develop skills from colleagues.

Partnership Work Is a Requirement, No Longer Optional

Fruitful partnerships in global mental health are now replacing older neo-imperialistic approaches to international work. Importantly, and rightly, this is likely to continue with strengthening of the principles of equality and mutual respect across the spectrum from humanitarian organisations (such as Médecins Sans Frontiéres), long-term bilateral part-nership-based organisations (such as Tropical Health & Education Trust) to global health institutes (such as the London School of Hygiene & Tropical Medicine). Working as volunteers now is *with* and *for* people in partnership with host countries, and increasingly everyone is learning from each other about how skilled, professional, culturally appropriate ethical care might look in the twenty-first century.

In Chapter 3, Dr Ayesha Ahmad questioned whether there are times when volunteers can do nothing that might be helpful. In doing so, the chapter gives cause for careful reflection about the motivations of volunteers and acts as a reminder to always keep the notion of not causing harm in the forefront of thinking at all times. The partnership model is particularly important as it allows for a process if things go wrong in individual programmes from the host's perspective – ranging from cultural appropriateness, personality clashes and systemic factors.

Professionalisation of Volunteering

Global volunteering is now moving on from the creative experimental phase of global mental health to real professionalisation of volunteers' work. Sometimes the best intentions, clinical knowledge and motivation are not enough. Volunteering in the future needs to be based on sound knowledge of global mental health and should follow some of the principles outlined in this book. These include human rights, sensitivity to culture and a public mental health perspective.

Global health volunteering is a privilege and it demands professionalism. This includes conducting a volunteering commitment with integrity and responsibility, and it should be done both ethically and sustainably. Chapter 4 considers a number of ethical challenges that may be encountered, and it is important that best practice is applied in the future. In particular, when witnessing unprofessional acts or behaviours by other volunteers, it is important that these are addressed swiftly. Increasingly, volunteers are not only representing themselves when working internationally, but also their sponsoring institution and profession. As such, it is key that all acts are professional and place the host community and related needs (and their definitions of professionalism) as central. Unprofessional behaviour during the voluntary placement can erode trust not only between individuals but also between the sponsor institution and host community, as well as wider professional groups.

Research and Evidence

There is growing recognition that goodwill and a trial-and-error approach is not enough. Voluntary work that involves interventions in training, clinical provision or service development needs to be evaluated and researched to identify and demonstrate what actually works to improve the mental well-being of the world's population. Robust evidence based on carefully planned and evaluated interventions can make a sustained difference to the resources and skills of health care workers and the health systems around them. The sense of being overwhelmed by the need to do something can become tempered by a realistic appraisal of what can usefully be contributed by volunteers.

The field of global mental health as an academic and research discipline is also significantly growing. Many colleagues who are motivated to volunteer globally are choosing to pursue research activities in this area, either complementary to or instead of voluntary placements. This is often done to further capacity building as part of institutional partnerships to encourage longer-term changes which ensure sustainability. In addition, such endeavours also seek to bridge the large research gap between high- and low-income countries, as historically most evidence has been generated by high-income countries.

Considering the role of research as important to the health and wealth of any nation, it is likely to be an important area for volunteers to help capacity build in the future – for example, around training with research skills, methodology and supervision.

Generational Shift in Attitudes

There has been, and there continues to be, a shift in attitudes to health practices and volunteering between generations, in both those volunteering and those hosting and receiving volunteers. There are now active efforts to ensure that colonial power relationships are not continued or furthered, and that any work undertaken is equitable, ensuring access and gender representation. Healthcare professionals around the world can increasingly express different attitudes, ideas and thoughts and it is likely that these may evolve in the coming years with a more vibrant, dynamic and younger health workforce owing to demographic transitions.

Personal and System Benefits of Volunteering

Many healthcare professionals are increasingly considering ways to engage in a portfolio career, characterised by undertaking a number of clinical and healthcare-related roles concurrently – for example, combining clinical work with being a teacher, researcher, advocate and volunteering in some capacity. Volunteering adds an extra dimension to the continuing development of becoming a good psychiatrist. Hopefully this will be increasingly recognised institutionally, and undertaken more widely.

National and international volunteering helps to move from personal focused preoccupations about how medicine and psychiatry (and life) works, to a broader perspective about the context of how most people in the world live, work, suffer and recover from mental ill health with the support of family, faith and community, as well as the interventions of health care professionals. As well as cognitively learning a great deal, volunteers can benefit from knowing that they have done something for others, without overt reward, and feel a satisfaction that can be hard to find in everyday UK practice. Seasoned volunteers report experiencing kindness, creativity and eagerness to learn and teach whilst working in global mental health, and express gratitude for the opportunity for personal development.

There is growing evidence that shows the value of mutual learning and benefits to the NHS as well as to the host country. Apart from the valuable experience of individual professionals undertaking a volunteering project, the UK overall benefits from learning creative and productive ways of managing mental health in low-resource settings.

Challenges – Some New, Some Continued

The transition from being a UK health worker within a relatively well-regulated NHS to working as an international volunteer can be challenging. Adaptability, team working, and good preparation help to make a safe and satisfying experience.

Other challenges to the work ahead for volunteers include difficulties in getting leave from work, funding issues and finding suitable, supportive and ethical placements. This can be particularly difficult as some training programmes in the United Kingdom are becoming more rigid and there are requirements to take 'out of training programme' years. This is something to monitor closely, and prospective volunteers may wish to plan voluntary placements alongside training opportunities. It remains preferable for psychiatrists to have a post graduate qualification in psychiatry such as a Member of Royal College of Psychiatrists before undertaking global mental health voluntary work and a natural opportunity may be between core and higher speciality training.

The barriers to mental health care in many countries remain huge. Mental health is often a low priority, with poor training for staff, frequent paucity or lack of psychotropic medicines and appropriate supervision. Substantial and sustained change takes time and volunteers need to have patience. Further, there continue to be systemic challenges. For example, brain drain to high-income countries will continue to be a constant concern and the presence of big pharma and gender inequalities need attention. The migratory pressures may worsen with climate change and other geo-political determinants.

Our role as volunteers is to be available to work with partners in ways that they find helpful, within their resources and culture. At present, and likely in the future, this is mainly through good mental health training and other supportive interventions.

Opportunities

Health workers should contact their professional bodies for further volunteering opportunities. Psychiatrists wanting to develop international projects in mental health can contact the volunteering programme of the Royal College of Psychiatrists. In Appendix 1 there is also a list of some of the opportunities and organisations to contact. There are also suggestions throughout of some useful books and articles, references and websites that have inspired previous volunteers.

Conclusion

As partnership working in global volunteering is evolving, it is necessary to approach voluntary experiences with an open mind, humility and a recognition and celebration of differences. While volunteering may often be daunting, difficult and unsettling at times, it is also exciting, fun, deeply rewarding and potentially transformative. Hopefully you will give it some serious thought, check out what is possible and give it a try by applying the principles outlined in the book.

We would like to express our gratitude to all the generous and hospitable people who have worked with the authors in this book to support volunteering and to improve the well-being of people with mental illness worldwide. We thank all those people living with mental health difficulties for inspiring us to write this book.

References

1. World Health Organization Academy. www .who.int/about/who-academy.

2. EQUIP (Ensuring Quality in Psychological Support). www.who.int/ teams/mental-health-and-substance-use/treatment-care/equip-ensuring-quality-in-psychological-support.

Appendix 1 Volunteering Opportunities

Global Voluntary Opportunities and Organisations

- Devnet – www.devnetjobs.org
- Doctors of the World UK – www.doctorsoftheworld.org.uk
- DSS – www.drrteam-dsswater.nl/mhpss
- Health Education England Global Health Exchange – www.hee.nhs.uk/our-work/attracting-recruiting/international-office/global-health-exchange
- Idealist.org – www.idealist.org
- International Medical Corps – www.internationalmedicalcorps.org.uk
- Jaya Mental Health – www.jayamentalhealth.org.uk
- King's Sierra Leone Partnership – www.kslp.org.uk
- King's Somaliland Partnership – www.kcl.ac.uk/aboutkings/strategy/profiles/Kings-Somaliland-Partnership.aspx
- Malawi Scottish Partnership – www.scotland-malawipartnership.org
- Médecins Sans Frontières – www.msf.org.uk
- Medical Aid – www.medicalaid.org/volunteer/mental-health/
- MHIN – www.mhinnovation.net
- MHPSS – www.mhpss.net
- Relief web – www.reliefweb.int
- Royal College of Psychiatrists, College Volunteer Scheme for Psychiatry Doctors – www.rcpsych.ac.uk/workinpsychiatry/internationalaffairsunit/volunteersscheme.aspx
- Royal College of Psychiatrists, VIPSIG – www.rcpsych.ac.uk/workinpsychiatry/specialinterestgroups/volunteeringandinternational.aspx
- Royal College of Psychiatrists' Volunteering and International Psychiatry Special Interest Group (VIPSIG) associated Facebook Page – www.facebook.com/groups/vipsig/
- Peter Hughes Twitter Account – @psychvolunteer
- THET Tropical Health Education Trust – www.thet.org
- Unity in Health – www.unityinhealth.org
- United Nations – www.unjobs.org
- The World Psychiatric Association (WPA) Volunteering Working Group (WG) – https://www.wpanet.org/wg-on-volunteering
- *Royal College of Psychiatrists' Volunteering and International Psychiatry Special Interest Group (VIPSIG) Associated Twitter Page -* @RCPsychViPSiG

Notable Research Global Mental Health Groups in the UK

Centre for Global Mental Health – King's College London and London School of Tropical Hygiene and Medicine – www.centreforglobalmentalhealth.org/

University College London – Global Mental health, www.ucl.ac.uk/mental-health/people/mental-health-researchers-directory/global-mental-health

Appendix 2 Practical Preparation Checklist

Health
- Travel consultation
- Vaccinations and vaccination card
- Malaria prophylaxis
- First aid kit
- Dental check-up
- Medical and hospital availability in country
- Physical fitness
- Psychological fitness

Insurance
- Travel insurance
- Medical indemnity

Risk Assessment
- Personal and professional

Paperwork
- Passport with 6 months validity as minimum and copies of passport details
- Visa/s
- Registration in country, if needed
- Letter of welcome from hosts
- Arrival details of person meeting you
- Address of accommodation
- Contact details of colleagues, hosts, family, own GP, bank
- Emergency plan (if something serious happens to you)
- Copies of everything important in print and in phone/s

Money
- Credit cards, including UK number for loss/theft
- Cash in local currency, if possible
- Cash in internationally acceptable currency, for example US dollars

Personal
- A good bag
- Suitable clothing for venue
- Bathroom needs
- Spare phone, loaded with photos of important information
- Water bottle
- Money belt, locks

- Torch
- Penknife
- Plug convertor
- Diary
- Entertainment/Kindle loaded
- Small 'can't live without'

Professional
- Laptop loaded with presentations
- Devices for connection to PowerPoint and outlets
- Powerpack for recharging devices
- Memory sticks, loaded with whatever might be needed
- Hard copies of essential books and handouts
- Gifts for hosts

Plan for Return Home
- Job, family, finances, debrief, reports

Glossary

Terms	Definition
ARCP	Annual Review of Competence Progression, what is used for annual review of progress of medical trainees in UK
Balint group	psychotherapeutic doctors forum
CB	Capacity building – this is the improvement of knowledge, skills and practice.
CRPD	Convention of the Rights of Persons with Disabilities – United Nations Treaty from 2006 that enshrines rights of disabled including mental illness. Signed by almost all countries of the world.
Foundation Doctor	In the UK the term for a doctor who qualifies before specializing.
FCDO	Foreign, Commonwealth and Development Office – UK government department that deals with all overseas matters.
FGM	Female Genital Mutilation – a common practice in many countries to cut and modify female genitalia for cultural reasons. This is against human rights.
GBV	Gender Based Violence – violence that is against women.
GMC	General Medical Council – body that regulates doctors in the UK.
HEE	Health Education England – NHS body in England.
HIC	high income country
IASC	International guidelines on mental health and psychosocial support in emergency settings. International guidelines on dealing with emergencies.
IMC	International Medical Corps. One of the leading iNGOs.
iNGO	International non-governmental organisation.
LMIC	Low- and Middle-Income Country – term for countries that are less developed according to the World Bank.
LSHTM	London School of Hygiene & Tropical Medicine – London-based research institution.
MGMH	Movement for global mental health
mhGAP	Mental Health Gap Action Programme – this is a WHO programme that supports increased delivery of mental health to people in LMICs through capacity building and task shifting of local health workers.
mhGAP-IG	Mental Health GAP Action Programme – Intervention Guide Version 2.
mhGAP-HIG	Mental Health GAP Action Programme – Humanitarian version.
MHIN	Mental Health Innovation Network – platform for mental health led by WHO and LSHTM.
MHPSS	Mental Health and Psychosocial Support – an approach that covers medical, social and psychological in dealing with patients.
NHS	National Health service
NGO	Non-governmental organisation – charitable organisations.

OCHA	United Nations Office for the Coordination of Humanitarian Affairs – this is the coordinating body in humanitarian emergencies of the United Nations.
OOPE	Out Of Programme Experience – time taken out by trainees in psychiatry from their training.
PFA	Psychological First Aid – a practical, supportive way of dealing with people in distress.
Protection	This is the action of keeping people safe from any harm. This relates to human rights violations of violence, rape, etc. There are national and refugee systems to ensure safety in accordance with international humanitarian, human rights and refugee laws.
PTSD	Post-Traumatic Stress Disorder – a type of stress disorder that occurs after severe life-threatening events.
RCPsych	Royal College of Psychiatrists – a professional charity that represents psychiatrists in UK
SDG	Sustainable Development Goals – these are international development goals. There are 17. Number 3 is on health.
Speciality Registrar Doctor	In the UK the term for a doctor in specialist training.
Task shifting	This is the principle where non-specialist health workers manage common and uncomplicated mental health problems.
THET	Tropical Health Education Trust – a UK-based charity that supports health and health system strengthening.
VIPSIG	Volunteer and International Psychiatry Special Interest Group – Royal College of Psychiatrists' group that promotes volunteering.
WHO	World Health Organization

Index

Printed in the United States
by Baker & Taylor Publisher Services